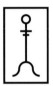

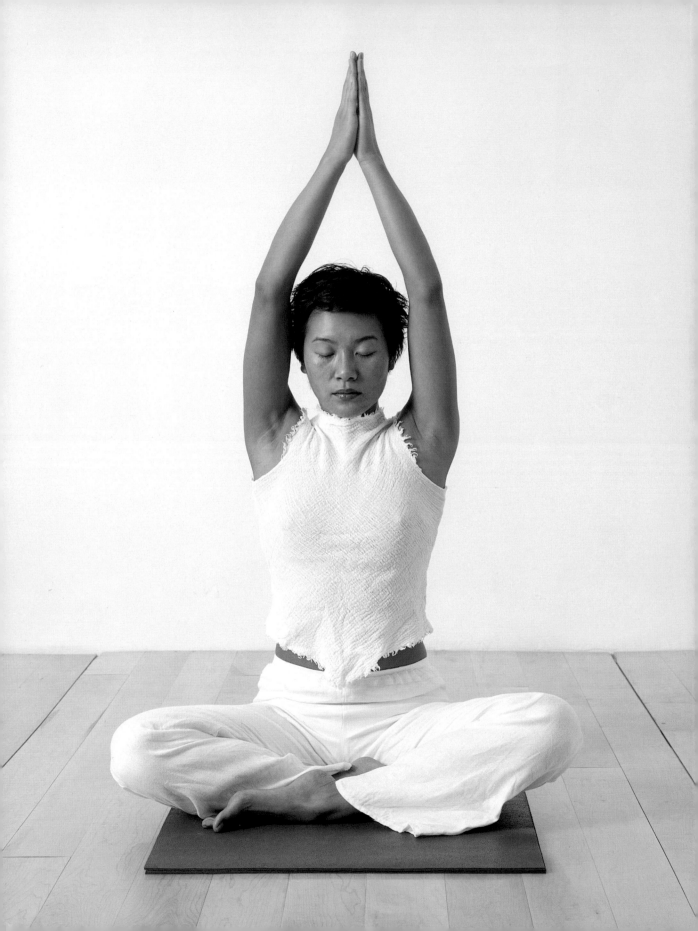

The
KUNDALINI YOGA
Experience

BRINGING BODY, MIND,
AND SPIRIT TOGETHER

GURU DHARAM S. KHALSA and DARRYL O'KEEFFE

A Fireside Book
Published by Simon & Schuster

New York London Toronto Sydney

This book is dedicated to Yogi Bhajan
whose ceaseless sharing of untold wisdom has made it possible.

———————————

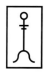

FIRESIDE
Rockefeller Center
1230 Avenue of the Americas
New York, NY 10020

For information about special discounts for bulk purchases,
please contact Simon & Schuster Special Sales:
1-800-456-6798 or business@simonandschuster.com.

Designed by Lucy Guenot

Printed and Bound in China by Toppan

10 9 8 7 6 5

Library of Congress Cataloging-in-Publication Data is available.

ISBN-13:   978-0-7432-2582-3
ISBN-10:   0-7432-2582-1

Foreword

As I traveled around the world with Yogi Bhajan from 1971 to 1987, and have traveled representing him since, I have personally encountered hundreds of thousands of people who have received comfort and upliftment from his teachings.

Being Yogi Bhajan's student/teacher is not easy. He never teaches in chapters, or in any order. It could be years before something he says in one lecture is clarified and expounded on in another. But being his student and a student of the teachings that he has shared gives a person grit, endurance, and the ability to be one-pointed, or to have mastery over the mind, which is the aim of meditation, as he puts it.

One doesn't just write a book about a spiritual practice without practice and experiencing some sort of inner results. Yogi Bhajan's students have to be eager and self-motivated to deeply go into his teachings to fully grasp the sacred science of Kundalini Yoga.

I have known Guru Dharam Singh Khalsa and Darryl O'Keeffe for over twenty years and have seen their perseverance in practice, and patience for learning. It is these very faculties that they themselves have achieved, as students of the teachings of Yogi Bhajan.

Guru Dharam and Darryl have gathered the material and have compiled it in such a way to simply explain the way to practice Kundalini Yoga based on the interconnection between the practice of the meditations and kriyas of Kundalini Yoga, the KY numerological system, the chakras, and the ten bodies. They have demystified the teachings, as well as distilling them into modern terms without sacrificing their purity. They have followed Yogi Bhajan's directive to be teachers themselves and have gone one step further to become teacher trainers and to finally write this book.

When we sat at the feet of the master in the 1970s and he talked about how each one of us has a destiny to fulfill, we could not then imagine how our destinies would manifest 30 years later. Guru Dharam and Darryl have served their destinies by sharing what they know has added quality to their lives with others. They do honour to Yogi Bhajan, their teacher.

Satsimran Kaur January 2002
Member of the Board of Directors 3HO Foundation
Member of the Board of Directors Kundalini Research Institute
Managing Director of White Tantric Yoga

Contents

About this book   **8**

Introduction
kundalini: the essence of yoga   **10**

Yogi Bhajan: a modern master   **15**

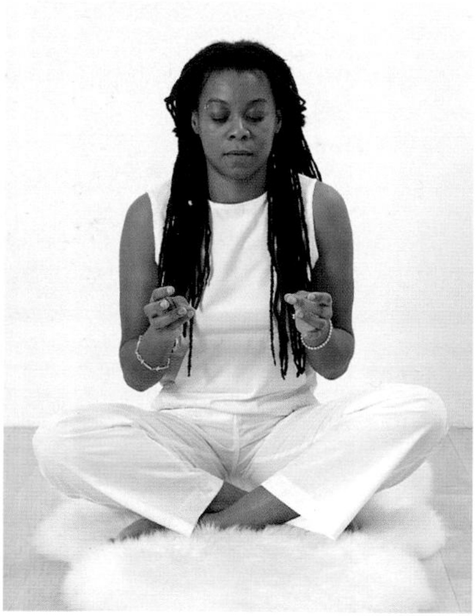

Part 1
you, your numbers, and your chakras   **16**

Yogic Numerology   **17**
Using the Numbers   **17**
What are Your Numbers?   **19**

1 The Soul Body   **21**
2 The Negative Mind   **22**
3 The Positive Mind   **23**
4 The Neutral Mind   **24**
5 The Physical Body   **25**
6 The Arc Line   **26**
7 The Aura   **27**
8 The Pranic Body   **28**
9 The Subtle Body   **29**
10 The Radiant Body   **30**
11 The Embodiment   **31**

The Chakra System   **32**
1st Chakra   **35**
2nd Chakra   **36**
3rd Chakra   **37**
4th Chakra   **38**
5th Chakra   **39**
6th Chakra   **40**
7th Chakra   **41**
Your Chakra Balance   **42**
The Chakra Questionnaire   **42**

Part 2
your practice   **50**

The Kundalini Yoga Experience   **51**
Your Personal Preparation   **52**

Part 3
the kriyas and meditations — 60

A Kriya and Meditation for Everyone for Every Day — 61

First Chakra MULADHARA — 64
Kriya for the First Chakra

Second Chakra SVADHISTHANA — 70
Kriya for the Second Chakra

Third Chakra MANIPURA — 78
Kriya for the Third Chakra

Fourth Chakra ANAHATA — 84
Kriya for the Fourth Chakra

Fifth Chakra VISHUDDHA — 88
Kriya for the Fifth Chakra

Sixth Chakra AJNA — 94
Kriya for the Sixth Chakra

Seventh Chakra SAHASRARA — 100
Kriya for the Seventh Chakra

Meditation for the Soul Body — 106
Meditation for the Negative Mind — 107
Meditation for the Positive Mind — 108
Meditation for the Neutral Mind — 109
Meditation for the Physical Body — 110
Meditation for the Arc Line — 111
Meditation for the Aura — 112
Meditation for the Pranic Body — 113
Meditation for the Subtle Body — 114
Meditation for the Radiant Body — 115
Meditation for the Embodiment — 116

Part 4
kundalini components — 118

Breath — 119
Mantras — 121
Mudras — 125
Asanas — 128
Bandhs — 134

Glossary — 136
Bibliography and resources — 138
About the authors — 140
Index — 141
Acknowledgements — 143

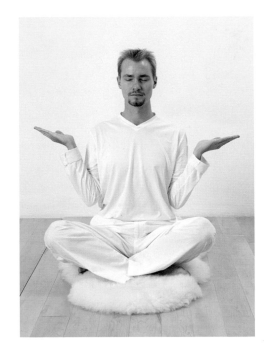

About this book

This book has been structured so that you can divine and develop a personalized programme of Kundalini Yoga over a number of years. It is not intended to be read from cover to cover and then banished to the bookshelf. Two main pathways help you decide which exercises will be of the most benefit to you, at the present time. One pathway is numerology, which enables you to work out your significant numbers and choose one aspect of yourself that needs attention. If, for example, numerology (see pp.17–20) shows you that you need to work on your Physical Body (see p.25), you choose a meditation for the Physical Body (see p.110). The other pathway is the chakra system. Using charts (see pp.35–41) and a questionnaire (see pp.43–9), you assess which chakra you need to give attention to and turn to the appropriate yoga exercise set, or kriya, for that chakra. For example, if your Third Chakra needs work, choose a kriya for the Third Chakra (see pp.78–83).

Kundalini Yoga kriyas and meditations work in many ways, on many levels. The metaphysical realities are understood by a Master, but their effects may be experienced by anyone. All the kriyas and meditations in this book were originally taught by Yogi Bhajan, the modern master of Kundalini Yoga. An experienced teacher of Kundalini Yoga may appreciate some of the ways in which the master has constructed the kriyas and some of the components from which the meditations have been created. The route to your own understanding is experience. We recommend that your practice, where possible, is supervised by a Kundalini Yoga instructor certified by KRI, the Kundalini Research Institute. There may not be a local teacher to guide your practice, answer your questions, and show the way forward and so we have tried to provide a means of determining which Kundalini Yoga practices may be particularly beneficial for you. This will help you towards understanding how and why they produce the effects that you will experience and instruct you in their safe practice.

This book is divided into four parts. Part One (You, Your Numbers, and Your Chakras) shows you how to learn about

Cautionary note
Consult your doctor before beginning this or any other exercise programme. Nothing in this book is to be construed as medical advice. The benefits attributed to the practice of Kundalini Yoga come from the centuries-old yogic traditions. Results will vary from one individual to another.

The word "God"
We have used the "G word" throughout this book. You do not have to believe in one specific god; any One will do and you are not excluded from these practices if you do not believe in any god. A spiritual technology will deliver no matter what you start out believing. Kundalini Yoga recognizes a spiritual totality; in essence all is One and we feel the word "God" conveys this concept most readily to most people.

"The One who Generates,
Organizes,
Destroys or Delivers
(G-O-D);
those are the three powers of God."
Yogi Bhajan 1996

yourself using numerology and the chakra system. Part Two (Your Practice) prepares you for practicing Kundalini Yoga, while Part Three (The Kriyas and Meditations) teaches you the yoga kriyas and meditations, giving detailed step-by-step instructions. Part Four (Kundalini Components) outlines important information about the separate techniques (the Breath, the Mantras, the Mudras, the Asanas, and the Bandhs) that make up Kundalini Yoga.

Do not try to do too much too soon. Do not force your body into something that it is not ready for. If you cannot sit in Lotus Pose, try Easy Pose; if you cannot sit on the floor, sit on a chair (keeping your spine straight and your feet on the ground). Do the best you can. This is all that you ask of yourself in Kundalini Yoga. Do your best. No one can do more. Others may go on for longer or go faster, but you can only do your best. Often you may not give your best; you hold back and keep a little in reserve. Don't let your mind tell your body that you cannot do something. You can do things that your mind might tell you are impossible. The exercises are usually short, so put everything you can into each one. If you were a short-distance runner and you did not put all your effort into your ten-second sprint you would achieve nothing. The same is true with Kundalini Yoga; what you get out is proportional to what you put in. You have to put in the effort and you have to keep up.

Concentrate on excelling. Respect the transformative power of Kundalini techniques. Do not attempt the maximum times suggested, however strong, fit, or flexible you are or you may trigger more subtle awareness than you are ready to integrate. Stick to the recommended structure and do not pick and choose what you do. The kriya prepares the body for the meditation. If you are too focused on the exercise itself you may miss the more subtle experience. Meditation is your dialling code to an aspect of your higher consciousness. Push the buttons exactly as instructed or you will get a wrong number. The result is assured, but only you can deliver it.

Special note for women

MENSTRUATION: *While bleeding do not practice Breath of Fire, navel pumping or any inverted postures.*
PREGNANCY: *Listen to your body and apply the following guidelines as your pregnancy progresses. Avoid postures and movements that strain the abdominal muscles, particularly backward bends. Avoid Breath of Fire (see p.120). Be cautious about forcing the body or overstretching, as the muscles and joints soften during pregnancy. Be aware that your sense of balance is changing. Look forward to mother-and-child yoga. As your own physical activities are restricted your child is beginning his or her own yoga practice within you.*

What to wear

From a quick glance at the pictures in this book, you will notice that all the models are wearing white and some are wearing turbans. Kundalini Yoga practitioners wear white cotton and natural fabrics to nurture the electromagnetic field. It is not essential to wear a turban, but you could try it. It will massage your cranial bones and focus your energy.

Introduction

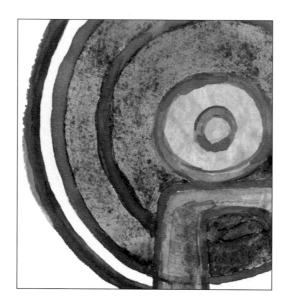

Kundalini: the Essence of Yoga

"Yoga" means "union" or "to yoke" in Sanskrit, describing the means for the Self to reunite with the whole. Every religion is a yoga in that each points to God, and every holistic practice is in essence a yoga in that it promotes the harmony of the whole. The postures commonly described as "yoga" make up but one of many yogic paths. "Kundalini" literally means "the coil in the hair of the beloved", but symbolizes the uncoiling of the inner awareness of our spiritual nature. Kundalini Yoga is the means by which we can safely prepare to activate and channel Kundalini energy, to raise our consciousness through the chakras, and through which we can transform our heightened spiritual awareness into constructive action. Kundalini Yoga is a powerful, transformative, spiritual technology; fast, focused, and effective. It is your birthright and the purpose of this book is to show you how to access it.

The first mention of yoga is circa 600BC in the Upanishads and earlier yogic practice, circa 2000BC, is depicted on seals found in the Indus valley, but it is reasonable to assume that its origins go further back. Ten thousand years ago weather shifts initiated extensive migration and such change must have produced renewed cultural stimulation and revised spiritual practices. Mythology ascribes the initial transmission of Kundalini Yoga to the god Shiva, who instructed his consort, Parvarti, in the sacred art. Yogic practice initially comprised Tantra, Laya, and Kundalini Yoga, each distinct, but together a trinity of ecstasy.

Kundalini is our latent spiritual potential, depicted as a serpent coiled at the base of the spine. This latent force is awakened by Kundalini Yoga as a psychic nerve energy. Its purpose is to raise consciousness, ascending via the chakras to the crown, connecting to the Infinite and realizing Samadhi (enlightenment). Attempting or achieving this process is "raising Kundalini". Bringing that awareness back down and applying it in the everyday world for the greater good is the less-talked-about completion of the Kundalini journey.

The three original yogic forms, Kundalini, Laya, and Tantra, were practiced by communities who celebrated and experienced infinite consciousness during the Sat Yug (the

The eight limbs of yoga

YAMA	self control
NIYAMA	observance of duty
ASANA	posture
PRANAYAMA	breath control
PRATYAHARA	inhibition or withdrawal of the senses
DHARANA	concentration
DHAYANA	meditation
SAMADHI	absorption in the Spirit

Golden Age of Truth, which ended 40,000 years ago). Over time, this *magnum opus* of yogic transcendence disappeared into the dark clutches of secret brotherhoods, innocent ignorance, deliberate obfuscation, religious avarice, and through "natural selection". The coherence of the yoga trinity gave way to deconstruction into constituent parts. There is no one definitive classification of the modern paths, but perhaps the three have become nine (see right).

The purification and preparation of the body for the earlier yogic disciplines began 1000 years ago to develop into the mastery of the postures, now known as Hatha Yoga, which most people understand as "yoga". Contemporary variations of yogic paths continue to multiply: from Ashtanga to Zen. Thus one unified sacred technology became the wellspring for all modern forms of yoga as recorded in the Vedas and in some cases as still practiced today. The arena for this dissemination was India, "the cradle of spirituality" of current civilization.

The pursuit and experience of Divine consciousness and the transcendence of the ego has always been a universal theme and the phenomenon of Kundalini undulates through our collective efforts to transform, elevate, and embody the truth of life. This was discovered by great mythologists and dreamcatchers; the work of Carl Jung and Sir James Gordon Fraser is redolent with tales of reverence for the serpent as teacher. Whether in the Caduceus, symbol of the medical profession, or in the twined double helix of DNA, the coiling and uncoiling of the serpent remains a potent point of global cultural reference.

Through time and space the ancient knowledge has percolated across cultures and down lineages, through royal houses, from teacher to student, and ultimately through the sound current of the Word, or the Logos. As the teachings perhaps attempted to protect themselves from the mundane world they sought refuge in the monasteries of Tibet: living in the hearts and minds of itinerant sadhus; in the glorious teachings of the Bodhisattvas; in the sacred texts of the Kabbalah; and in the Koans of the Zen Masters. As we

The nine modern paths of yoga

BHAKTI	*the yoga of devotion*
HATHA	*the yoga of the body*
JNANA	*the yoga of wisdom*
KARMA	*the yoga of service*
KUNDALINI	*the yoga of latent spiritual awareness*
MANTRA	*the yoga of sound*
RAJA	*the yoga of the mind*
TANTRA	*the yoga of sexual polarity*
YANTRA	*the yoga of vision*

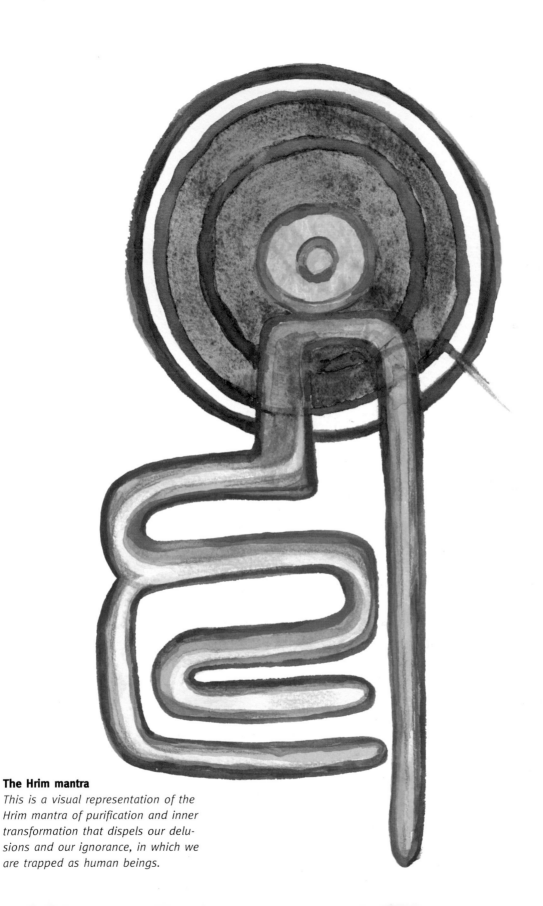

The Hrim mantra

This is a visual representation of the Hrim mantra of purification and inner transformation that dispels our delusions and our ignorance, in which we are trapped as human beings.

attempt to shift our consciousness into an Aquarian mode of pluralist, inclusive, and universally compassionate heartspace, the re-emergence of Kundalini Yoga represents an invaluable and authentic source of transformation for all.

Yogic Energetic Physiology

The purpose of raising Kundalini energy is to achieve Samadhi, to experience the full energy of consciousness or the energy of full consciousness. The Kundalini process fuses the energies of Shakti, the female principle, with Shiva, the male principle. Through practice of Kundalini Yoga the pranic force is directed downwards, as the apanic force is directed upwards, using the Mul Bandh and Uddiyana Bandh (see Bandhs, pp.134–5). This generates powerful psychic heat called Tapa. These forces are mixed at the Navel Point in an alchemical fusion of Shakti and Shiva energies. This energy is directed to penetrate the Base (First) Chakra, around which dormant Kundalini energy lies coiled. This initiates the awakening of Kundalini, which rises through the central Sushumna. If the channels of Ida and Pingala are clear, and the intent of the aspirant is pure, Kundalini can rise, activating each chakra, and realizing Samadhi. The ability to maintain or access this union gives spiritual liberation and is the fully awakened Kundalini. Kundalini energy is like a rocket; it may eventually transcend gravity, but its tendency is to be aroused, to rise up, and then fall back into its sleeping state.

The path of rising Kundalini is blocked if the Bandhs (see pp.134–5), or body locks, are not in place, or if one or more chakras are blocked. These are the causes of the physical, emotional, or mental disturbance experienced by those in whom rising Kundalini is triggered prematurely. The practice of Kundalini Yoga progressively removes their causes and is increasingly used in a variety of therapeutic modalities. Even with regular practice energy is unlikely to rise initially to the Crown (Seventh) Chakra. Benefits lie in regular, sustained practice and are measured in subsequent improvements in the quality of life.

Yogi Bhajan: a modern master

History will remember Yogi Bhajan as the person who gave authentic Kundalini Yoga to the modern world, breaking the centuries-old code of secrecy and elitism that had shrouded this practice. When Yogi Bhajan came to the West in 1969 he clearly stated his intention: "I have come to create teachers not to gather disciples". He has created thousands of teachers since then who are at the heart of an international community called 3HO, the Healthy Happy Holy Organization, which supports, practices, and spreads the teachings.

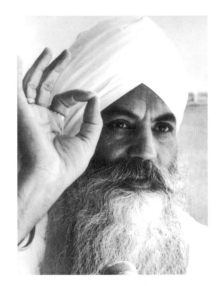

Yogi Bhajan was born Harbhajan Singh Puri in 1929, in India. His spiritual tutelage began at seven years of age and at 16 his teacher, Master Sant Hazara Singh, pronounced him Master of Kundalini Yoga. At the age of 18 he led 1000 people through the turmoil of partition to safety in Delhi after their village became part of Pakistan. He received a Masters degree in Economics from Punjab University, where he excelled both in the debating chamber and on the athletics field. He then established a successful career, serving in the Tax and Customs Division of the Indian Government before he was invited to the West. In 1953 he married Bibi Inderjit Kaur and they have three children and five grandchildren.

Although he is recognized as a seer, sage, healer, philosopher, business and religious leader, Yogi Bhajan is primarily a spiritual teacher with a global constituency. His work is published in over 200 books and videos and he received a PhD in the Psychology of Communication in 1980. Yogi Bhajan holds three major spiritual offices. He has defined the role of Director of Spiritual Education of 3HO. He is also known as the Mahan Tantric, directing the practice of White Tantric Yoga around the world, after the title and office was bestowed on him in 1971. Yogi Bhajan is also known by the Sikh community as the Siri Singh Sahib, since being invited to become the Chief Religious and Administrative Authority for Sikh Dharma in the Western hemisphere in 1971.

Yogi Bhajan has been lauded and lambasted. He has found and lost fame and fortune. As a yogi he is at home in all circumstances and with all people, sharing, inspiring, and teaching, with infinite love and humour, the technology of coexisting in the Age of Aquarius as elevated, radiant beings.

Part 1

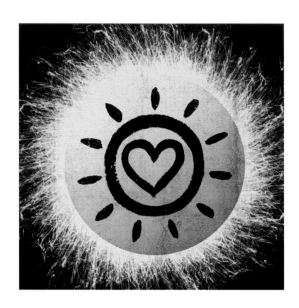

you, your numbers,
and your chakras

Yogic Numerology

Throughout the ages the significance of birth dates has been recognized by diverse cultures. Today we celebrate our birthdays and are intrigued by our horoscopes (derived from the relative positions of the planets currently and at the time of our birth). We might conjecture that the tides are pulled by the Moon and that humans are largely constituted of water, so more distant planetary objects could exert a subtle pull on us. A spiritual technology cannot be fully comprehended at the lower vibratory levels of the mind. The tree is known by its fruit: a spiritual master is known by his truth. Yogi Bhajan has shared this simple process by which we may prepare for the challenges and opportunities offered to us in this lifetime and revealed to us through our date of birth.

The Ten Bodies and the Eleventh Embodiment

All is one. Everything is in its essence the same. The frequency at which something vibrates determines its nature. We are souls having a human experience and journeying back to the Source; seeking to align to the essence within and without being distracted by all that lies between. Our **Soul** (first stage, see p.21), is journeying through the aspects of the human psyche: the ten yogic bodies. After conception our soul emerges from the Infinite within and becomes conscious of, and surrounded by, thought. Thought comprises the **Negative Mind** (second stage, see p.22) and the **Positive Mind** (third stage, see p.23), which as a whole produce the **Neutral Mind** (fourth stage, see p.24). The soul and mind (or minds) find expression in the **Physical Body** (fifth stage, see p.25). The progression of the soul requires the support of mind and body. The **Arc Line** (sixth stage, see p.26) guides the way on for the soul. The **Aura** (seventh stage, see p.27) is the flow of electromagnetic energy within and around the physical body. It interrelates with the seven chakras and is the space through which we hold or release past experience. The **Pranic Body** (eighth stage, see p.28) fuels spiritual growth, connecting us to the prana, or Life Force (chi, ki, or qi). The **Subtle Body** (ninth stage, see p.29) is the next

Using the Numbers
Work out what your five yogic numbers — Soul, Karma, Gift, Destiny, and Path — are (see pp.19–20) and then use them to discover which energy body you need to work on by reading the number charts that follow, on pp.21–31. If, for example, you find that you need to work on your Physical Body, you then turn to the meditation for the Physical Body (p.110) and incorporate that into your daily Kundalini Yoga practice.

vehicle of the soul, through which it leaves the physical, but before that journey is taken it is the means through which we tune in to the subtle flow. The **Radiant Body** (tenth stage, see p.30) is our spiritual radiance, our innocence. It is that which our soul aspires to and as our soul journeys through the other bodies it finds the radiant body in each. The **Embodiment** (see p.31) is the point from which the soul and radiant body, reunited, perceive all that has been between. It is the sum that is greater than the whole of the parts.

Calculating and Using the Numbers

Using the chart on the following pages (19–20) calculate your five numbers, each between one and 11. You may have five different numbers or you may have some repeats. Each one relates to one or more of your subtle bodies and the position of that number is a clue to the inherent state of balance of that body. Now reveal your life path by turning to the appropriate section (Soul, Karma, Gift, Destiny, and Path) under each of your five numbers. How well have you met the challenge in each position? If you are not manifesting the balanced aspect of a body you will, by default, be manifesting its negative counterpart.

Having read the five sections relevant to you, decide which yogic body you need to work with now and turn to that number in Part 3 (see p.60). If you do not feel you have accomplished the Soul challenge start there, making that your first step. If you feel you have done so consider whether claiming your Gift could help in your Karmic challenge and make one of these your second step, the other your third step. Your fourth step will be the Destiny Number, your fifth step will be the Path Number. Don't rush. We all get there in the end. You have identified the yogic bodies most relevant to you, but remember we all have a full set of 10 + 1 yogic bodies and work with them throughout our yoga practice and our life. The objective in this section is to point to a particularly beneficial meditative practice for you at this point in your life.

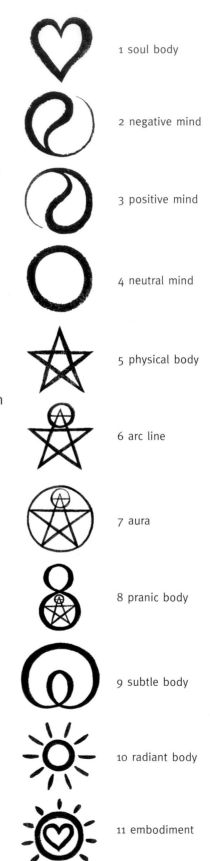

1 soul body

2 negative mind

3 positive mind

4 neutral mind

5 physical body

6 arc line

7 aura

8 pranic body

9 subtle body

10 radiant body

11 embodiment

What are Your Numbers?

Conventional numerology deals only with single numbers. Double digits are added together to reduce them to a number between 1 and 9. Therefore 23 will reduce to 5 (2+3) or 20 will reduce to 2 (2+0). Classical numerology refers to certain other significant numbers, which point to a spiritual insight and which should not be reduced, such as 11 and 22 (the double 1 and double 2).

The system taught by Yogi Bhajan reduces every number above 11 and relates it to one of our ten yogic bodies or to the eleventh, the Embodiment. Therefore 19 or 28 will reduce to 10 (not 1) and 29 will reduce to 11 (not 2).

Let us now calculate your yogic numerology.

Soul Number

Your Soul Number is the day number of the date you were born on.

For example:
If the day of your birth is between the 12th and 31st, add the two digits together to give you a number between 1 and 11. For example, 15 reduces to 6 (1+5). If you were born on the 15th your Soul Number is 6.

If the day of your birth is between the 1st and 11th, you already have your Soul Number.

The Soul Number represents the first challenge in your life, to make connection between your inner and outer self (or between your Higher Consciousness and your everyday awareness). Until you make this connection you are lost in a world to which you can only relate physically, emotionally, or mentally. When you connect to your soul consciousness you become aware of yourself as more than body and mind; the awareness of soul establishes you as a spiritual being. Once we become secure in our inner connection to our spiritual nature we have unshakeable inner strength. This is something most people achieve over time. Wisdom comes with age: the techniques in this book will help you to smoothly overcome life's challenges.

Karma Number

Your Karma Number is the month number of the date you were born.

For example:
If the month of your birth is 12, add 1+2 to give you 3.
If your month of birth is between 1 and 11 you already have your Karma Number.

The Karma Number represents the second challenge of your life, which can only be met once you have achieved the first. Once you have connected to your soul truth and raised your individual spiritual standard you have to hold to your truth in the face of the challenges of those around you. It is relatively easy to connect to your spiritual nature in peace and seclusion. It is somewhat harder to maintain that connection in the face of external disruption. The challenge of the Karmic Number, then, is to speak your truth and walk that talk.

Gift Number

Your Gift Number is the sum of the last two digits of the year in which you were born.

Add together the last two digits of the year of your birth and reduce it to give you a number between 1 and 11.

For example:
1979 reduces to 7 (7+9=16, 1+6=7). For those born in 2000, count the 00 as 10.

The Gift Number is not a challenge, it is a birthright. It is a talent, an opportunity that you are offered in this lifetime to assist you on your spiritual journey. It is a gift, but you have to claim it, develop it, and honour it (use it or lose it).

Destiny Number

Your Destiny Number is the sum of all the digits of the year of your birth.

For example:
1979 reduces to 8 (1+9+7+9=26, 2+6=8).
For those born in 2000, the number is 2 (2+0+0+0=2).

The Destiny Number need not be a challenge, but it may seem to be. It has been said that our destiny is written on our forehead, but this is a very difficult place for us to see it. Consequently our destiny is reflected to us by those around us. This can mean that you are the last to recognize the truth that everybody else has always known about you. Our Destiny Number represents the skills our soul has mastered in the past. It is how other people see us. It is how we are rather than how we think we are. The challenge is for us to see ourselves as others see us and follow the destiny we have already charted for ourselves.

Path Number

Your Path Number is the final sum of adding together all the digits of your birth date.

For example:
If you were born on 6/5/1961 your path number is 10 (6+5+1+9+6+1=28. Then 2+8=10).

If you were born on 12/11/1977 your path number is 11 (1+2+1+1+1+9+7+7=29. Then 2+9=11).

If you prefer, add together your Soul, Karma, and Destiny numbers (but not the Gift Number as this is contained in the Destiny Number).

The Path Number is your path to fulfillment in this lifetime. All your other numbers contribute to your path, so do not neglect to develop them. Your Path Number is the sum of your parts. Your final challenge is for the whole to exceed the sum of the parts.

1 The Soul Body

All is One

The Soul is the Traveler and the Journey. In our Soul Body we listen to the Infinite and through our Soul Body we convey the Infinite knowing into the finite world around us. The Soul is the Divine aspect of our Self, our Higher Self, which follows the steps of our evolutionary journey from union through separation to reunion as One. When we connect to our soul we consciously awaken to our journey; we become co-creators with God.

To balance this body, turn to the meditations on page 106.

Number 1 in the Soul Position

When this body is unbalanced you will be self-centered and lost in your thoughts. Your inner conflict is between head and heart. As long as the head dominates you will often feel unhappy and the outcome will be unsatisfactory because deep inside you know things are not what they might have been. Your challenge is to harness your intuition and your intellect and to find creative expression in the balance between the two.

Number 1 in the Karma Position

When this body is unbalanced you will be dependent, stubborn, inflexible, and manipulative. You need to be creative to be yourself; your outer need is to express your inner originality. Your inspiration comes not from the head but from the heart. When this body is balanced you will relate to other people at the level that feels comfortable to your inner self and not at the level that you think that they may find appropriate.

Number 1 in the Gift Position

When this body is unbalanced you will be unstable and self-centered. When you claim this gift you will be confident, soulful, and able to give innovative expression to your latent creativity.

Number 1 in the Destiny Position

Your soul's journey has shown you all the positive and negative aspects of this body. Others will value you for your positive and original contributions, which will be sought by them more often than offered by you. If you do not recognize this description of yourself you need to balance this body.

Number 1 in the Path Position

Your path in this lifetime is to inspire others through your originality and creativity; to express your soul self and, in so doing, to be a living example to others that to "be yourself" is a balanced, constructive contribution to the whole. When this body is balanced you know, and those around you remember, that we are all One.

2 The Negative Mind
Longing to Belong

The separation of one from the whole abandons the one into the duality of the two. The negative mind is the second stage of our soul-conscious journey; learning who we are by defining who we are not. The negative mind reveals every route to "no" and in so doing points out every pitfall before "yes". When we connect to our Negative Mind we acquire the discernment to move on safely.

To balance this body, turn to the meditations on page 107.

Number 2 in the Soul Position
When this body is unbalanced you will long to belong. This inner longing needs a spiritual discipline, or teaching, and you will be over-emotional until you become devotional. Balance this body, become secure in yourself, and prepare to consciously seek and follow your spiritual path.

Number 2 in the Karma Position
When this body is unbalanced you will be antagonistic and unrealistic. You will try to be all things to all people and may have a succession of empty and failed relationships. The need to be needed will supplant the discernment to select and receive what you really need for your soul growth. Loyalty in a relationship and unforced chastity outside of one are indicators of balance in this body.

Number 2 in the Gift Position
When this body is unbalanced you will be pessimistic, irritating, and easily irritated because you are unable to hold your own space. When you claim this gift you will become secure in your energetic space and respectful of the space of others.

Number 2 in the Destiny Position
Your soul's journey has shown you all the positive and negative aspects of this body. You are recognized by all as thoroughly sensible and valued as a loyal friend. You are noted for your skill in handling people and as a natural mediator. If you do not recognize this description of yourself you need to balance this body.

Number 2 in the Path Position
Your path in this lifetime is to recognize and commit to following the spiritual path that is calling you. The "divine marriage" is your assured route to fulfillment. Listen to your soul and when it resonates with the path before you, commit. Rather than longing to belong, long to be. Choose to bring the inner longing into outward expression.

3 The Positive Mind

I Will, to Will, Thy Will

In the third stage of our soul-conscious journey, having defined what we are not, we now discover what we can be. The Positive Mind sees the positive aspect in any situation. It is our enthusiasm and it needs our support and encouragement or it will be negated. If we do not use the Positive Mind its default position will be to reinforce the Negative Mind. Once we dwell in the Positive Mind we rise to the challenge of the world around us. Anything is possible and nothing can stand in our way, but in our enthusiasm we may not consider whose will we are imposing upon whom.

To balance this body, turn to the meditations on page 108.

Number 3 in the Soul Position

When this body is unbalanced you will experience shades, or even the extremes, of self-doubt or self-certainty. The latter will prove to be unfounded as long as it derives from your personal will rather than the greater Will and consequently increases your self-doubt and decreases your self-worth. Until you see God in all, you have not seen God at all.

Number 3 in the Karma Position

When this body is unbalanced you will negate yourself. You will be hesitant and uncertain and others will easily manipulate you. Even when secure within your own power you may fear the consequence of using it and this is a sure route to losing it, as the positive mind will defer to the negative. Until you can see God in all, you cannot see God at all.

Number 3 in the Gift Position

When this body is unbalanced you will be unable to appreciate yourself. You may be given to brooding, self-doubt, and depression. When you claim your gift you will find the confidence to express your true self and realize the ability to see the positive side of everything.

Number 3 in the Destiny Position

Your soul's journey has shown you all the positive and negative aspects of this body. Others will be attracted to your company, recognizing you as helpful, fun to be with, and counting on you to point to the positive viewpoint in any difficulty. If you do not recognize this description of yourself you need to balance this body.

Number 3 in the Path Position

Your path in this lifetime is to practice and encourage positivity in all and equality for all. Always look on the bright side of life and encourage others to do the same through your example and constant good humour. Smile, you know God loves you, and you, and you...

4 The Neutral Mind
Beyond Duality

Having appreciated the extremes of positive and negative we try to find a balance between the two; in so doing we begin to detach ourselves from the world of duality, of opposites, of extremes, but in balancing two extremes we remain attached to both. The Neutral Mind is a state of non-attachment and is the fourth stage of our soul-conscious journey. It is an integration of opposites into one, rather than a balance between two. The Neutral Mind accepts the input from all our other bodies, integrates it, and offers us guidance. When you don't know what to do or say count to ten and allow the Neutral Mind the nine seconds it needs to review the input from all your other bodies and guide you. The Neutral Mind measures value, not in cost but in truth.

To balance this body, turn to the meditations on page 109.

Number 4 in the Soul Position
When this body is unbalanced you will be indecisive. You will see things from many different perspectives, but will be lost among them and unable to select one viewpoint to act upon. This may lead you to become close-minded, even dogmatic, as you avoid the confusion of choice. When this body is balanced you will see those different perspectives as aspects of a whole and will be certain of your position in relation to them.

Number 4 in the Karma Position
When this body is unbalanced you will be unable to keep your opinions to yourself. You will tend to be dogmatic and argumentative. You may even enjoy argument for the sake of it. Even when you can utilize the Neutral Mind in your own decision-making you will be unable to accept that those close to you need the space to do the same. When this body is balanced you are able to move beyond this duality and accept that everything outside of your control is as it should be.

Number 4 in the Gift Position
When this body is unbalanced you will tend to appear narrow-minded and judgmental, but you will be fundamentally indecisive and out of touch with yourself. When you claim your gift you will find that wisdom informs your decision and compassion serves as your motivation. You will see life's lessons revealed in every blessing or reversal of fortune. Your gift is to know that life itself is a gift.

Number 4 in the Destiny Position
Your soul's journey has shown you all the positive and negative aspects of this body. You have a generous nature and are able to see the practical reality behind the drama. You will be seen as open-minded by others and they will value your wisdom and insight into life and the lessons it teaches us. If you do not recognize this description of yourself you need to balance this body.

Number 4 in the Path Position
Your path in this lifetime is to exercise compassion. You are a peacemaker. Preach what you practice; promote integration by revealing to all the underlying unifying structure in any representation of duality or separation. Help others to find value in their experience and truth in their values.

5 The Physical Body
Teacher of Balance

Five is the number of the teacher and this teacher is taught by life. The Physical Body is the fifth stage of our soul-conscious journey. It is the space in which all the other bodies play out their interaction through the medium of life, action, and circumstance. Here the balance is struck between the upper (spiritual) and lower (physical, emotional, and mental) worlds. We may choose to indulge the senses on the physical plane indefinitely, but eventually following the spiritual path of evolution will be the only new experience left to us. At any time we can consciously choose to reduce the wait.

To balance this body, turn to the meditations on page 110.

Number 5 in the Soul Position
When this body is unbalanced you will be fundamentally out of balance at the center of your being and this can permeate into any and every aspect of life. You will have an uneasy relationship with your Physical Body and may tend towards being a hypochondriac. You will be attracted to opposite extremes. You will see the whole in both, but being unable to be in both simultaneously you will swing from one to the other. Your momentum will be such that you will be moving fastest as you pass through the point of balance between. Your strategy to cope may be inertia, which may manifest as laziness. When this body is balanced you will know the still point at the center of a storm of activity.

Number 5 in the Karma Position
When this body is unbalanced you will be unable to balance the conflicting needs of yourself and others. You will find it particularly difficult to put the needs of others before your own and if you do so it will be as a martyr. You may be secretive and reluctant to share what you know. When this body is in balance you will tend to have good health and will feel healthy. You will also have the personal discipline to make sacrifices for the good of others.

Number 5 in the Gift Position
When this body is unbalanced you will not be comfortable with your Physical Body and will tend towards laziness and indulgence. You will be uncommunicative within yourself and towards others. When you claim your gift you will manifest health, generosity, and self-discipline and will, in one way or another, become a teacher or communicator.

Number 5 in the Destiny Position
Your soul's journey has shown you all the positive and negative aspects of this body. You are comfortable with your appearance and have an easy relationship with your body. You have a natural sense of balance and an inborn grace and athleticism. You love to share. You are a natural communicator and teacher and will invariably be looked to by others as such. If you cannot recognize this description of yourself you need to balance this body.

Number 5 in the Path Position
Your path in this lifetime is simply to share what you have, know, and are: to teach, both by personal example and by utilizing your God-given communication skills. You are able to find the point of balance at the center of anything; now find yourself as a teacher of balance.

6 The Arc Line

Power to Project through Prayer

The sixth stage of our soul-conscious journey lights the way home. The Arc Line does not belong to the world through which we have so far moved; it is the base of the Radiant Body and manifests in the everyday world through the power of prayer. It has been depicted through the ages as the halo around the head of a saint, and indeed is most visible as a 6–9-mm (2–3-in) arc from earlobe to earlobe. Women have an additional line between the breasts, but for each one of us the Arc Line, visible or not, passes through the whole body. The Arc Line is not subject to the laws of nature; it is governed by a higher realm. It gives us the power to project and manifest our own reality. Its radiance protects our positive being and deflects our negative projections, whether they come from within or without.

To balance this body, turn to the meditations on page 111.

Number 6 in the Soul Position

When this body is unbalanced you will avoid the use of your intuition and will busy yourself with the ways of the mundane world. You will be unable to concentrate on the task in hand and will generally lack focus and direction. You may tend to find yourself in the wrong place at the wrong time. When this body is balanced your intuition will be sharp, you will have a strong inner direction and an uncanny ability to be in the right place at the right time.

Number 6 in the Karma Position

When this body is unbalanced your focus will be easily disturbed by others. You will be easily caught up in their dreams or delusions. You will find it hard to set goals and even harder to achieve them. You may find yourself accident-prone. When this body is balanced you will be a success story. You will do what you say you will do and you attract the opportunities to manifest your expressed intentions.

Number 6 in the Gift Position

When this body is unbalanced you will be unable to focus your concentration and will be out of touch with your intuition. When you claim your gift you will begin to manifest your own reality; this is a two-edged sword. You have the power to create your negative reality as well as your positive one; be careful what you wish for.

Number 6 in the Destiny Position

Your soul's journey has shown you all the positive and negative aspects of this body. You have always had a strong inner-soul connection and maintain a regular practice of prayer or meditation. Others see you as being able to take a dream and make it real. You are recognized as someone who gets things done, in the best possible manner and in the way that most honours all. If you cannot recognize this description of yourself you need to balance this body.

Number 6 in the Path Position

Your path in this lifetime is to be guided by your meditation practice. Listen to the still, silent voice. Contemplate its guidance and act upon it in the manner that best honours all. The meditation may be in the moment, but always meditate before your initial action.

7 The Aura

Raising your Vibration

The seventh stage of our soul-conscious journey is through the auric field in which past and future is played out. The Aura is created by the flow of prana through the nadis or meridian lines of the body and the interaction of the chakra system. It is a sphere of electro-magnetic energy, which can extend for up to 2.75 m (9 ft) beyond the physical body. The Aura holds the memories of our past experience, which can act as karmic ties and hold us back. The Aura also offers us a secure space, beyond our physical body, through which we attract the grace to grow and into which we move our consciousness as we realize our existence beyond our physical dimensions.

To balance this body, turn to the meditations on page 112.

Number 7 in the Soul Position

When this body is unbalanced you will lack the inner security and confidence to move forwards. You will be unable to trust anything new and will withdraw into yourself. You will tend to dwell on the failures of the past. Your immune system may be weak and you will tend to catch whatever is going around. When this body is balanced you will feel good about yourself. You are absolutely certain who you are and where you are going.

Number 7 in the Karma Position

When this body is unbalanced you will be prey to all manner of energetic disturbance around you and will be unable to distinguish between that which is caused by you and that which is caused by others. You may be so caught up in your inner world that you are unable to relate to groups of people. When this body is balanced you will be fearless. You are able and willing to be, but you will not need to be, the center of attention and the life and soul of any party.

Number 7 in the Gift Position

When this body is unbalanced you will repel rather than attract. When you claim your gift you manifest a magnetic personality that positively attracts and uplifts. Your security comes not from what you have, or think you have, but from knowing who you are. You are at home wherever you are because you are at home with yourself.

Number 7 in the Destiny Position

Your soul's journey has shown you all the positive and negative aspects of this body. You are totally secure within yourself and consequently have the capacity to exhibit infinite patience and tolerance towards others. You have charisma; there is a certain aura about you. People enjoy just being with you. You are the stranger in the street people stop and ask for directions; you are both approachable and inspirational. If you cannot recognize this description of yourself you need to balance this body.

Number 7 in the Path Position

Your path in this lifetime is to attract and inspire others towards practices that develop their awareness of their own energetic space. You will find fulfillment in sharing your personal experience of the expression of unconditional love and the practice of mercy.

8 The Pranic Body

Resurrection

The eighth stage of our soul-conscious journey resurrects our consciousness of prana. The Pranic Body connects us to the Life Force of Infinity and distributes that energy throughout the finite aspects of our being. Throughout life we breathe; the first and last thing we do in life is to breath in. Oxygen is the fuel burned by the cells; prana is the fuel burned by the Life Force that constructs those cells. The source of prana is infinite, but our capacity to access it is finite. A yogi lengthens his life by breathing more slowly; as we master prana we begin to master life and to develop the capacity to move beyond death.

To balance this body, turn to the meditations on page 113.

Number 8 in the Soul Position

When this body is unbalanced you may lack energy and you will lack staying power. You may sleep too much and rely on shortcuts to energy such as sugar or caffeine. Over time your weakness will lead to fearfulness. You are particularly prone to worrying about lack of money. When this body is balanced you have boundless energy, need little sleep, and are not afraid to try anything.

Number 8 in the Karma Position

When this body is unbalanced you will tend to be over-cautious, even defensive, in your interactions with others. You will have the desire to succeed, but will lack the application to plan and follow through with your ambitions. When this body is balanced not only will you have the energy to implement your intentions but you will also transmit this energy and enthusiasm to those around you.

Number 8 in the Gift Position

When this body is unbalanced you will be lacking in energy and prone to addictive behaviour. When you claim your gift you connect to unlimited reserves of energy. You are able to energize those around you. If you do use up all your energy you can recharge your batteries in a short space of time.

Number 8 in the Destiny Position

Your soul's journey has shown you all the positive and negative aspects of this body. You have boundless energy. You seem to attract wealth and respect. You have a natural ability to energize those around you and may be recognized as a healer. If you cannot recognize this description of yourself you need to balance this body.

Number 8 in the Path Position

You are a natural healer. Your path in this lifetime is to uplift and heal others through sharing your energy and enthusiasm for life. Through your example others, too, can resurrect their tired bodies and minds and reconnect to the infinite flow of pranic energy.

9 The Subtle Body
Master of Mystery

The ninth stage of our soul-conscious journey brings us to the Subtle Body through which our soul will move after leaving our physical body. All the intricacies of the worlds around us are known through this body. The Akashic Record (see p.136) may be read here; our subconscious nature is written on this body. Thus far on our journey it is as if we have seen one different tree after another. Now, for the first time consciously, we can see the wood in which the trees are growing and with this insight we become masters of what seemed unfathomable mysteries a moment before.

To balance this body, turn to the meditations on page 114.

Number 9 in the Soul Position
When this body is unbalanced you will only recognize opportunities after they have passed you by and you may have a tendency to be clumsy. You will never be able to satisfy your curiosity, will tend to be over-analytical and suffer from information overload. When this body is balanced you will have the grace to know without thought, the sensitivity to perceive the structure beneath, and you will never be deceived by surface appearance.

Number 9 in the Karma Position
When this body is unbalanced other people mystify you; you never know where they are coming from and you will be blissfully insensitive to their sensitivities. You will be easily taken in and deceived. You may be too easily diverted and will rarely finish anything because you will already have started something else. When this body is balanced you will be in tune with the world around you and will pick up the subtle clues that put you into the flow of awareness.

Number 9 in the Gift Position
When this body is unbalanced you will be clumsy and insensitive and may find yourself disturbed by psychic energy or awareness. When you claim your gift you will be able to tune in to the essence of anything. You will pick up new skills quickly as you seem, somehow, to have done it all before. You know, before anything is said.

Number 9 in the Destiny Position
Your soul's journey has shown you all the positive and negative aspects of this body. You have mastered your chosen field. You have the capacity to see beyond form and to know the unknown. You are naturally intuitive and express yourself artistically with grace and subtlety. If you cannot recognize this description of yourself you need to balance this body.

Number 9 in the Path Position
Your path in this lifetime is to utilize your natural mastery of the subtle realm to smooth the way onto the path for others. Your chosen field may be artistic or humanitarian, but whatever field you choose, use your gifts to help others master their mystery by reflecting what is, not what it appears to them to be.

10 The Radiant Body
Hero to Zero

Ten is the number from which all things have sprung and into which they must return. The tenth stage of our soul-conscious journey brings a conscious reunion with the Light. At every stage of the journey the soul has been drawn to the Light; now, once more, it immerses itself in It. Yogi Bhajan refers to this number as 1+, the soul of 1 plus the infinite o of our God-given radiance. Where there is light there can be no darkness. When we are one with our Radiant Body the impenetrable radiance reflects any external negativity and neutralizes any internal negativity within a 2.75-m (9-ft) space of our physical body. The glow of that radiance can subtly promote harmony across a 40-km (25-m) radius.

To balance this body, turn to the meditations on page 115.

Number 10 in the Soul Position
When this body is unbalanced you will feel overwhelmed. You will be unable to motivate yourself. You may have an ongoing identity crisis as you avoid owning up to your power. When this body is balanced you radiate benevolent power. You are unshakeable.

Number 10 in the Karma Position
When this body is unbalanced you are unable to sustain an effort under pressure. You will avoid challenges and give way even when in the right. When this body is balanced you will stand firm for what you believe in. Your word will be your bond. You are unstoppable.

Number 10 in the Gift Position
When this body is unbalanced you will be unreliable, untidy, and un-noticed. When you claim your gift you will attract attention and command respect. You will stand out by your courage, your commitment, and your continued effort long after others have given up.

Number 10 in the Destiny Position
Your soul's journey has shown you all the positive and negative aspects of this body. You have an unshakeable inner strength and a powerful and inspirational presence. You are prepared to stand up for what you believe in regardless of the consequences. If you cannot recognize this description of yourself you need to balance this body.

Number 10 in the Path Position
Your path in this lifetime is to be as a saint. Raise your spiritual standard as high as you can and live up to it; accept nothing less than your best. God loves you and through you.

11 The Embodiment
Equilibrium

We have come to the completion of our soul-conscious journey. Beyond lies Infinity; in due course we will tread that path. Here in the Embodiment we have consciousness of all ten of our bodies of light. We are able to understand and direct their interaction. We are our own spiritual master. We see all the choices in every option and we choose God because it is our only option. We have reached equilibrium in our Self and now we choose to maintain and extend that equilibrium in our interaction with others, because we understand that we are all One.

To balance this body, turn to the meditations on page 116.

Number 11 in the Soul Position
When this body is unbalanced you will value the material world over the spiritual and will tend to have too high an opinion of yourself. When this body is balanced you will commit yourself to one spiritual technology or teaching and practice it with humility and dedication.

Number 11 in the Karma Position
When this body is unbalanced you will be reacting to situations rather than positively influencing them. You may tend to interfere in the business of others. You will taste one spiritual practice after another, but will not sustain the spiritual discipline. When this body is balanced you will commit yourself to one spiritual technology or teaching and practice it with humility and dedication.

Number 11 in the Gift Position
When this body is unbalanced you will be materialistic, inflexible, and reactive. When you claim your gift you will grow to be humble, compassionate, and able to flow positively into any moment or situation with grace and effectiveness.

Number 11 in the Destiny Position
Your soul's journey has shown you all the positive and negative aspects of this body. You are conscious of the interplay of your ten yogic bodies. You have attained spiritual mastery of yourself. If you cannot recognize this description of yourself you need to balance this body.

Number 11 in the Path Position
Your path in this lifetime is to be a living demonstration of conscious collaboration with God. Manifest your spiritual mastery of your ten yogic bodies in all your thoughts, words, and deeds.

The Chakra System

It is often said that prayer can move mountains. If we believe in a subtle energy, like prayer, or if we have experienced its effects upon our physical body, such as in Kundalini Yoga, we may ask, "What makes this possible?" Could such a mechanism be beyond our comprehension? The most widely adopted model to explain this is the chakra system. "Chakras" may be translated as "wheel" and depicted two-dimensionally, but they are perhaps better described as spinning vortices of energy existing in many dimensions. It is in using them as tools for insight that their greatest value lies. The chakra system is a model through which we can make sense of life. The existence of chakras cannot be proven, but as a theoretical model they have stood the test of time and are interpreted primarily in three ways:

1. As a process of evolution

We can observe our progress through life. First we had to explore our physical body. Secondly our emotions. Thirdly we formed a mental image of the world. These three steps may be represented as a growing up of our consciousness through the lower chakras: First Chakra (physical), Second Chakra (emotional), and Third Chakra (mental). As a species we have yet to evolve beyond conscious control of our lower three chakras. The upper chakras comprise the spiritual centers: the Fifth, Sixth, and Seventh Chakras. The integration of upper and lower chakras takes place at the Fourth Chakra.

2. As a transformer of energy

Energy healing is well documented, but it still eludes scientific explanation. The chakra system allows us to conceive that a subtle energy, such as prayer or love, can enter our consciousness through the chakras and effect change at a physical level, influencing hormonal secretions through interaction with nervous plexus and endocrine glands. This might seem far-fetched, but the remarkable correlation between the locations of the seven chakras and the endocrine glands is a fact. The endocrine system is fundamental to our well-being and the process by which it regulates itself is yet to be fully explained.

Using the chakras
These spinning "wheels of energy" are models that can give us insight into our true selves. Use the chakra charts on the following pages (pp.34–41 and pp.43–9) to help you decide which chakras you need to work on now. Then turn to the chakra kriyas on pp.64–105 to choose the right Kundalini Yoga exercises for you. There is a choice of two kriyas for each chakra.

The perceived physical location of the roots of the chakras also corresponds to various nerve plexes.

3. As a system of esoteric instruction

A third view maintains that the chakras have no existence in physical reality, but are merely focal points for our concentration; gateways beyond our physical state, through which we may eventually evolve into a new reality.

We can no more prove the existence of the chakra system than we can weigh the energy of love, but our consciousness provides the means to experience them. Each chakra resonates to a different frequency. Just as sunlight may be refracted into the colours of the rainbow, each chakra resonates to a different refraction of the Infinite Light. Red light has a slower vibration, bends least, and corresponds to the First Chakra, which has the slowest vibratory rate of the seven chakras. Violet is refracted the most and corresponds to the Seventh Chakra, which has the highest vibratory rate.

The material world relates to the lower chakras (First to Third) and occasionally the Fourth. The Seventh Chakra accesses energies beyond the everyday world. These higher vibratory rates are ever-present everywhere, but we are unable to sustain our consciousness of them until we can relate to the vibratory rate of each of our seven chakras. Vibratory rates are communicable and until you can manage your energetic space you will be disturbed. The people closest to you will affect you most: people with lower rates will pull you down, while people with higher rates will uplift you. The easiest way to raise your rate is to be with people who have already done so, but this will not prepare you to sustain that higher vibration when challenged by those who have not. However, regular Kundalini Yoga practice can soon render that a problem of the past.

We all have favourite colours; in the same way each of us relates more to one chakra than another. The following pages outline correspondences for each chakra and describe how a person primarily centered in each one will be. Consider which chakra you have primarily operated from at different times. Our vibratory rate is always changing, but there will be certain frequencies we return to because of unfinished business there, as we resist the changes that come with moving on.

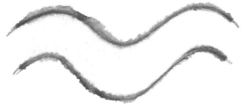

Slow vibrations

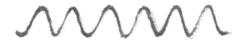

Higher vibration

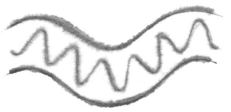

Higher vibration within lower vibrations

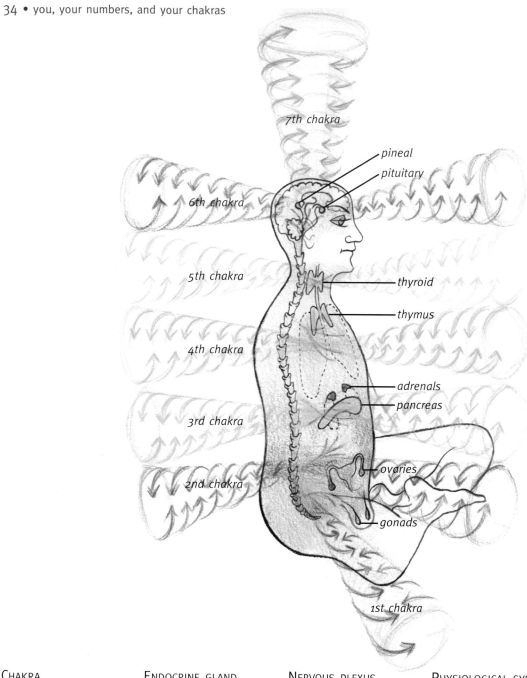

7th chakra

pineal

pituitary

6th chakra

5th chakra

thyroid

thymus

4th chakra

adrenals

pancreas

3rd chakra

2nd chakra

ovaries

gonads

1st chakra

CHAKRA	ENDOCRINE GLAND	NERVOUS PLEXUS	PHYSIOLOGICAL SYSTEM
1 • Muladhara	Adrenal	Coccygeal	Excretory
2 • Svadhisthana	Gonads/ovaries	Sacral	Reproductive
3 • Manipura	Spleen/ Pancreas	Solar	Digestive
4 • Anahata	Thymus	Heart	Circulatory
5 • Vishuddha	Thyroid/Parathyroid	Pharyngeal	Respiratory
6 • Ajna	Pituitary	Hypothalamus	Autonomic nervous
7 • Sahasrara	Pineal	Cerebral cortex	Central nervous

1st Chakra

The First Chakra is the foundation of the system. It relates to the Earth element and all solid Earth things. This chakra is involved with our bodies, our health, and survival (both primal and material existence). It relates to our ability to project, focus, and manifest our worldly, Earthly needs.

The person centered in this chakra needs to feel safe. They will be fundamentally insecure until their basic physical needs have been met.

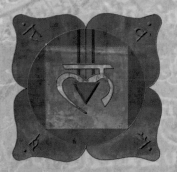

CORRESPONDENCES

Descriptive verb • *I have*
Force • *gravity*
Sense • *smell*
Food • *protein*
Element • *earth*
Colour • *red*
Celestial body • *saturn*
Creature • *elephant*

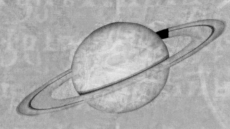

Physical • *constipation, haemorrhoids, obesity, sciatica, lower back pain*
Emotional • *fear, calm*
Mental • *self-awareness*

Sanskrit name
MULADHARA
meaning root or foundation

Other names
Root or Base Chakra

Physical location
The perineum, at the base of the spine

Nervous plexus
Coccygeal

Endocrine gland
Adrenals

Body associations
Bones, feet, immune system, large intestine, legs, rectum

KEY WORDS
Basic needs, grounding, security, survival

When this chakra is unbalanced/blocked it can manifest as:

- *Addictive behaviour*
- *Avoidance of intimacy*
- *Consideration of oneself regardless of others*
- *Distrustful or hostile relationship to the world*
- *Tunnel vision*
- *Workaholism, driven by a lack of self-worth*

When this chakra is balanced/unblocked it can manifest as:

- *Allowing oneself to be vulnerable*
- *Asking what can be learned from adversity*
- *Being in the present moment*
- *Trusting in God*
- *Valuing oneself*

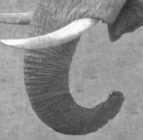

2nd Chakra

The Second Chakra is to do with Change. One becomes two, solid becomes liquid, and we immerse ourselves in the element of water. The consciousness of this chakra derives from flow, duality, and the attraction of opposites.

The person centered in this chakra needs the freedom to be creative. They will tend to indulge their desires.

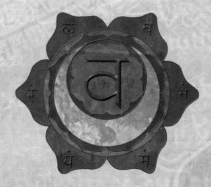

CORRESPONDENCES

Descriptive verb • *I feel*
Force • *magnetism*
Sense • *taste*
Food • *liquids*
Element • *water*
Colour • *orange*
Celestial body • *moon*
Creature • *crocodile, fish*

Physical • *frigidity, impotence, pelvic or lower back pain, urinary problems*
Emotional • *possessiveness, expansiveness*
Mental • *self-respect*

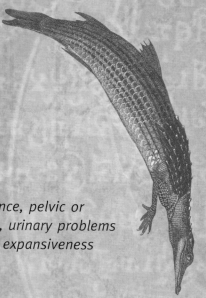

Sanskrit name
SVADHISTHANA
meaning sweetness

Other name
Sacral Chakra

Physical location
The sacral spine

Nervous plexus
Sacral

Endocrine gland
Gonads

Body associations
Bladder, genitals, kidney, large bowel, prostate, uterus

KEY WORDS
Creativity, desire, sexuality

When this chakra is unbalanced/blocked it can manifest as:

- *Exhibitionism*
- *Inadequacy*
- *Shallow relationships*
- *Shame of the body or sexuality*
- *Wild-child behaviour into adulthood*

When this chakra is balanced/unblocked it can manifest as:

- *Ability to initiate*
- *Empathy with others*
- *Generosity and a willingness to share*
- *Genuine intimacy*
- *Mutually empowering relationships*
- *Passion for life*

3rd Chakra

The Third Chakra has Fire as its element and with it comes choice, action, vitality, and will. In this chakra we explore personal power; is it to empower oneself or is it to have power over others?

The person centered in this chakra needs to achieve something and make their way in the world. They will utilize their own will to manipulate or inspire others in order to do so.

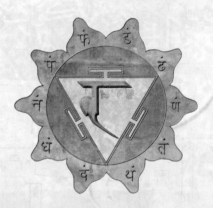

Sanskrit name
MANIPURA
meaning lustrous gem

Other name
Navel Chakra

Physical location
Navel/solar plexus

Nervous plexus
Solar plexus

Endocrine gland
Pancreas

Body associations
Digestive system, liver, muscles

KEY WORDS
Power, will

CORRESPONDENCES

Descriptive verb	• *I can, I do*
Force	• *combustion*
Sense	• *sight*
Food	• *carbohydrates, starches*
Element	• *fire*
Colour	• *yellow*
Celestial body	• *the sun*
Creature	• *goat, ram*
Physical	• *diabetes, hepatitis, indigestion, ulcers*
Emotional	• *anger, guilt, passion, trust*
Mental	• *self-worth*

When this chakra is unbalanced/blocked it can manifest as:
- *Dogmatic conformity*
- *Greed*
- *Need for external validation*
- *Rights over responsibilities*
- *The end justifies the means*
- *What's in it for me?*

When this chakra is balanced/unblocked it can manifest as:
- *Awareness of the effect of one's actions upon others*
- *Control over one's life*
- *Exemplary leadership skills*
- *Practicality*
- *What's in it for us?*
- *Will power*

4th Chakra

There is balance in all things: the expansiveness of air and the unconditional nature of love. When this center is unbalanced you will give to those who do not deserve it and share with those who do not want it.

The person centered in this chakra will be concerned with balance and finding the middle way or the natural rhythm. They will be motivated by love.

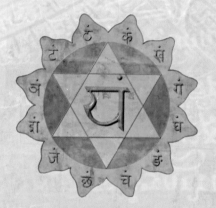

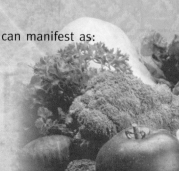

CORRESPONDENCES

Descriptive verb • *I love*
Force • *equilibrium*
Sense • *touch*
Food • *vegetables*
Element • *air*
Colour • *green*
Celestial body • *venus*
Creature • *antelope, deer, dove*

Physical • *asthma, circulatory system*
Emotional • *bitterness, grief, joy, love*
Mental • *self-love*

Sanskrit name
ANAHATA
meaning unstruck

Other name
Heart Center

Physical location
Center of the chest

Nervous plexus
Heart

Endocrine gland
Thymus

Body associations
Arms, hands, heart, lungs

KEY WORDS
Compassion, love

When this chakra is unbalanced/blocked it can manifest as:
- *Alienation*
- *Attachment*
- *Grief*
- *Loneliness*
- *Passive aggression*
- *Questioning the existence of love*

When this chakra is balanced/unblocked it can manifest as:
- *Acceptance that all is as it should be*
- *Harmonious relationships*
- *Harmony with nature*
- *Positive neutrality*
- *Seeing God in all*
- *Unconditional love for all*

5th Chakra

At the Fifth Chakra sound reverberates into the Ether. Purification is our purpose; communication is our focus; mantra and the vibration of sound our tools.

The person centered in this chakra will be resolving aspects of communication within themselves and towards others. They need to, and are able to, express themselves.

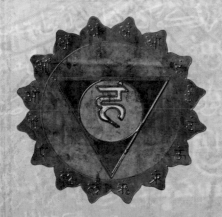

CORRESPONDENCES
Descriptive verb • *I communicate*
Force • *vibration*
Sense • *sound*
Food • *fruit*
Element • *ether*
Colour • *blue*
Celestial body • *mercury*
Creature • *cat, lion*

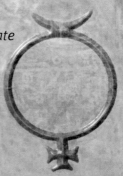

Physical • *ear, nose, and throat problems*
Emotional • *courage, frustration*
Mental • *self-expression*

Sanskrit name
VISHUDDHA
meaning purification

Other name
Throat Chakra

Physical location
Throat

Nervous plexus
Pharyngeal

Endocrine gland
Thyroid, parathyroid

Body associations
Neck, shoulders

KEY WORDS
Communication, creative expression

When this chakra is unbalanced/blocked it can manifest as:
- *Cunning*
- *Creative untruthfulness (deceit without lying)*
- *Frustration at inadequate communication*
- *Withdrawal from the emotions into the mind*
- *Shyness*
- *Speaking too bluntly*

When this chakra is balanced/unblocked it can manifest as:
- *Always voicing the truth*
- *Being listened to as an authoritative voice*
- *Hearing what has not been said*
- *Inspirational communication*

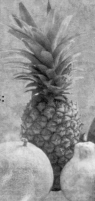

6th Chakra

We see what we expect to see; let there be light and let us see through darkness. Let us perceive the realms beyond as we transcend time and look beyond duality.

The person centered in this chakra will see things differently. They have inner sight and will find clarity wherever they focus.

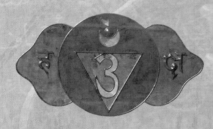

Sanskrit name
AJNA
meaning perception

Other name
Third Eye

Physical location
Center of the head projecting forwards between the eyes through the root of the nose

Nervous plexus
Hypothalamus, autonomic nervous system

Endocrine gland
Pituitary

Body associations
Eyes

KEY WORDS
Intuition, perception, sixth sense, vision

CORRESPONDENCES

Descriptive verb • *I perceive, I see*

Force • *psychic*

Sense • *intuition*

Food • *fasting or in some cultures certain hallucinogenic plants, usually now classified as poisons*

Element • *light*

Colour • *indigo*

Celestial body • *jupiter*

Creature • *owl, unicorn*

Physical • *eye problems, headaches, nightmares, sinusitis, visions*

Emotional • *clear, calm, confusion, inadequacy*

Mental • *self-responsibility*

When this chakra is unbalanced/blocked it can manifest as:

- *Being "out of it"; out of the body, or out of touch with the body.*
- *Confusion of what is real and what appears to be real*
- *Hiding in intellectual analysis (denial of actual experiential reality)*
- *Inability to focus on any one thing*
- *Psychic disturbance*

When this chakra is balanced/unblocked it can manifest as:

- *Being comfortable in any reality*
- *Clear perception*
- *Psychic abilities, particularly clairvoyance*
- *Reliable intuition*
- *Seeing energy within, and beyond, matter and form*

7th Chakra

In the Seventh Chakra we are all One. Every element of every chakra we have explored already is here. This is the chakra of knowing, and thought is the densest level of consciousness present.

The person centered in this chakra will know the unknown and be conscious of the Infinite. They will have experienced a reality beyond the realm of the physical senses.

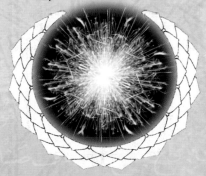

Sanskrit name
SAHASRARA
Meaning infinite

Other name
Crown Chakra

Physical location
Center of the head projecting up through the anterior fontanel

Nervous plexus
Cerebral cortex, central nervous system

Endocrine gland
Pineal

Body associations
Brain, nervous system

KEY WORDS
Divine knowledge and understanding, acceptance, bliss

CORRESPONDENCES

Descriptive verb • *I accept, I know*

Force • *consciousness*

Sense • *divine*

Food • *fasting*

Element • *thought*

Colour • *violet*

Celestial body • *uranus*

Creature • *human being* (There is no traditional association, but you might meditate upon a seed growing up from the Earth through your body and opening as a thousand-petalled lotus flower floating upon the crown of your head.)

Physical • *apathy, alienation, close-mindedness, symptoms without physical cause*

Emotional • *bliss, despair, doubt, joy, peace*

Mental • *self-consciousness*

When this chakra is unbalanced/blocked it can manifest as:

- *Abuse of "lower" life forms (human imperialism)*
- *Doubt and denial of the spiritual reality*
- *Religious extremism*

When this chakra is balanced/unblocked it can manifest as:

- *Bliss; being in but not of this world*
- *The experience of all as one*
- *The integration, expression, and actualization of such peak experiences*
- *Saintliness*
- *Samadhi*

Your Chakra Balance

This section is to help you choose your Kundalini Yoga kriya for today, by helping you discern which chakra is most out of balance, or blocked. The chakra charts (see pp.35–41) give an impression of how a person operating predominantly from one chakra seems, but you cannot discuss one chakra in isolation. All chakras interact with all others and each constantly changes. We can also come from one chakra through another. For example the Fifth Chakra facilitates communication, but the truth often hurts, so the blunt truth of the Fifth Chakra may be expressed through the Fourth; truth with compassion. Our world is predominantly in the image of the Third Chakra. Humankind is currently evolving from the Third to the Fourth. By the time you are mature you have had the chance to master your first three chakras. But there will be unfinished business in each and this should be an ongoing process, to be periodically readdressed. You will not have mastery of the upper chakras, but you can access and utilize them to assist your path of personal and spiritual growth.

The Chakra Questionnaire

Chakras are described as "open" or "closed", "unblocked" or "blocked", but it is really our consciousness of the chakra that is referred to, not the chakra itself. It is clearer to think of the changes in a chakra's state as energy spinning faster or slower, raising or lowering its vibratory rate. There is an optimum state for a chakra to be in, relative to the others and to our state of consciousness. The questionnaire statements (see pp.43–9) reveal whether each chakra is spinning faster or slower than optimum. Choose the most appropriate description for each issue and add the total for each chakra (3 = first column, 0 = second, and 1 = third). Compare your totals for each of the seven chakras. The chakra with the highest score is the one to work on today. Turn to pp.64–105 and select either kriya for that chakra. Practice this kriya for at least a week before reassessing. Record your findings and your Kundalini Yoga experiences for future review.

How do I discern which chakra I should work on today?

• *Read the chakra charts (see pp.35–41) and see if it is obvious which chakra you most resonate with.*
• *Use the Chakra Questionnaire (see pp.43–9) to assess which chakra you might address today.*
• *Access your intuition. If you are still unclear which chakra to work on, ask for guidance from your Higher Self and roll a die twice. The first number you roll is the chakra you should work on today (First to Sixth Chakras = 1–6), unless the second number you roll is the same (e.g. 3 and 3), in which case you work on the Seventh Chakra.*

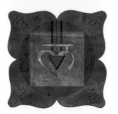

1st chakra

	Score 3	Score 0	Score 1	YOUR SCORE
1a	*You always seem to have an ache, a pain, or a bug of some sort*	*You enjoy consistently good health and shake off any minor ailments very quickly*	*Your health is generally excellent, with occasional collapses in which your seemingly good health is wiped out for days*	
1b	*You are well above or below your optimum weight, or do not know what it is*	*You are comfortable with your body and are at your optimum weight*	*You are reasonably close to your optimum weight*	
1c	*Your diet is poor or you do not know what a good diet for you might be*	*You know that you eat a balanced, healthy diet*	*You are overly concerned with your dietary needs*	
1d	*You are in considerable debt or are unable to use the excess of funds you have acquired*	*You have no financial worries or needs. Money flows easily and you always have enough for your needs*	*Money is attracted to you, but you never have enough*	
1e	*You are so spiritually aware that you are no Earthly use*	*Everyone sees you as a horoughly practical, down-to-Earth person*	*You tend to focus on the material world, to the exclusion of the spiritual*	
1f	*You rarely exercise*	*You maintain a regular, balanced exercise routine*	*You are obsessed with exercise*	
1g	*You have no particular interest in the natural world*	*You regularly make time to be in nature*	*You find it difficult to be away from the natural world*	

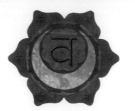

2nd chakra

	Score 3	Score 0	Score 1	YOUR SCORE
2a	*You are out of touch with your emotions*	*You are able to express your emotions when appropriate*	*You are unable to stop expressing your emotions*	
2b	*You have no sex life to speak of*	*You enjoy an active sex life*	*You are preoccupied with sex*	
2c	*You are unable to nurture others*	*You are able to support and encourage growth in others*	*You are unable to stand back and let others discover for themselves*	
2d	*You are unaware of the "flow"*	*You are able to "go with the flow"*	*You are lost in the "flow"*	
2e	*You are physically inflexible*	*Your body balances strength and flexibility*	*Your body is flexible, but you lack strength*	
2f	*You are emotionally inflexible*	*You are comfortable with all your emotions*	*You experience emotional swings*	
2g	*You rarely make time to relax or to enjoy yourself*	*You always find time to relax and enjoy yourself*	*You can never get enough pleasure*	

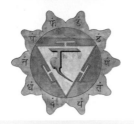

3rd chakra

	Score 3	Score 0	Score 1	YOUR SCORE
3a	Others manipulate you	You are aware of, and comfortable with, your personal power	You are manipulative of others	
3b	You lack self-confidence	You are always justifiably confident	You tend to be over-confident	
3c	You are often unable to achieve your goals	You always set and achieve reasonable goals	You tend to set and strive for unrealistic goals	
3d	You lack willpower	You choose when to apply your will	You tend to be over-assertive	
3e	You tend to avoid responsibility	You shoulder your responsibilities	You tend to feel you are responsible for everything	
3f	You never seem to have enough energy	You always have enough energy for your needs	You have too much energy and may have difficulty resting or sleeping	
3g	You rarely do what you say	You say what you can do	You do what you say, come what may	

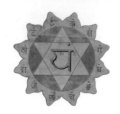

4th chakra

	Score 3	Score 0	Score 1	YOUR SCORE
4a	*You often feel depressed and sad*	*You always feel happy and content*	*You can be ecstatic, but swing quickly from happy to sad*	
4b	*You feel nothing is right*	*You feel all things are as they should be*	*You feel everything is perfect*	
4c	*You find it difficult to make friends*	*You are able to make and keep friends easily*	*You have many friends, but few close ones*	
4d	*You have maintained few long relationships*	*You have several significant long relationships outside your immediate family*	*None of your long relation- ships is deep or meaningful*	
4e	*You are uninvolved with the world around you*	*You are a part of the world around you*	*You feel yourself above the world around you*	
4f	*You are often unable or unwill- ing to experience compassion*	*Compassion moves you to empathy*	*Compassion usually dictates your actions*	
4g	*You are often unwilling to give or share*	*You are able to give and share freely*	*You often give to those who don't need or want*	

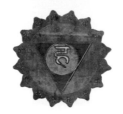

5th chakra

	Score 3	Score 0	Score 1	YOUR SCORE
5a	You are often unable to express yourself satisfactorily	You are able to express yourself appropriately	You tend to express yourself accurately and bluntly	
5b	You find it difficult to listen to others	You are able to hear what someone is trying to say	You often interrupt because you hear what has not been said yet	
5c	You have difficulty being creative	You are constructively creative	You tend to be indulgently creative	
5d	You do not like the sound of your own voice	You are comfortable with the sound of your own voice	You are too taken with the sound of your own voice	
5e	You are unable to focus on several ideas at once	You are able to synthesize different opinions in a group	You confuse others by holding several different points of view at once	
5f	You have few creative pastimes	You have several creative outlets	You have an overwhelming need to be creative	
5g	You do not have many good ideas	You put your best ideas into action	You have so many good ideas yet implement so few	

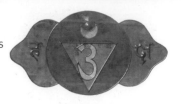

6th chakra

	Score 3	Score 0	Score 1	YOUR SCORE
6a	You are unable to trust your intuition	You are able to access and utilize your intuition	You tend to be overly reliant upon your intuition	
6b	You refuse to acknowledge psychic phenomena	You have accepted psychic phenomena as a natural part of your world	You tend to prefer the extra-ordinary to the ordinary explanation	
6c	You cannot recall your dreams	You recall and consciously reflect upon your dreams	You often have difficulty distinguishing between dreams and reality	
6d	You are unable to see your spiritual path	You see God in all	You do not value the spiritual paths that you do not follow	
6e	You do not think about the quality of light	You prefer natural light	You are uncomfortable in artificial light	
6f	You have a poor visual sense	You have a heightened visual awareness	You are overly reliant upon your visual perception	
6g	You prefer dull colours	You appreciate all colours but usually prefer to wear light shades	You are often drawn towards or wear overly bright colours	

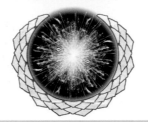

7th chakra

	Score 3	Score 0	Score 1	YOUR SCORE
7a	*You know that you do not really know yourself*	*You have spent time getting to know and like yourself*	*You do not really appreciate anything else beyond yourself*	
7b	*You have difficulty meditating*	*You meditate regularly*	*Your meditation practice often makes you late for appointments*	
7c	*You tend to act without consideration of the consequences*	*Your actions are guided by your meditative practice*	*You rarely initiate action*	
7d	*You rarely analyze anything*	*You reflect upon an issue or action and learn from it*	*You are over-analytical of your actions*	
7e	*You do not go into anything in great depth*	*You research everything thoroughly*	*You immerse yourself in unnecessary detail*	
7f	*You have not experienced anything you would describe as spiritual*	*You have integrated one or more profound spiritual experiences*	*You have no real interest apart from spiritual experience*	
7g	*You have no clear concept of God*	*God is with you*	*You are with God*	

Part 2

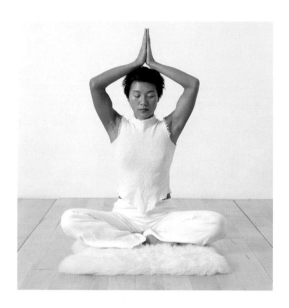

your practice

The Kundalini Yoga Experience

The best way to experience Kundalini Yoga is with a group of like-minded people under the direction of an experienced teacher. We have listed teacher associations in the Resources section (see p.139), but it is not always possible to find a suitable class and even if it is we hope you will still develop a regular personal practice. The object of this book is to provide you with all the information to pursue a safe and transformative personal practice.

Yoga is a Sanskrit word and is sometimes translated to mean yoke or harness. You are working with a powerful transformative spiritual technology and need to be aware of the appropriate guidelines for effective and safe practice. We know that a razor blade in the wrong hands is dangerous, yet every day millions of people use safety razors without harming themselves. Power is potentially dangerous unless it is safely harnessed. Follow the seven simple steps described on the next few pages to structure and enhance your Kundalini Yoga experience.

How long should I do this practice?

• *The day on which you can perform the exercises for the maximum specified time counts as Day One.*

• *Continue the kriya for 40 consecutive days to improve negative traits relating to the purpose of the practice.*

• *Continue for 80 days to implant a new positive habit pattern.*

• *Continue for 120 days to seal it in your psyche. Then choose another kriya.*

• *When you find the kriya that is your key to this lifetime, practice it for 1000 days, for self-mastery.*

• *Most benefit will be derived from your practice if it can be done at the same time every day. Why not rise before dawn, when your time is your own, and make this practice your morning Sadhana (see p.137)?*

Your Personal Preparation

The natural arena for yoga practice is your creation, or rather the re-creation, of a sacred space on both an internal and external level. Your body is a temple of consciousness and should reflect your intention to cleanse, heal, and uplift yourself and others in all things.

Set your energy for the day or for your yoga practice by having an invigorating cold shower. Oil your body with almond oil and vigorously massage yourself while enjoying the stream of water cascading over you. Pay particular attention to the feet and hands, as the 72,000 nadis (see p.137) all end there.

Wear white cotton and natural fabrics to nurture your electromagnetic field. It is recommended that you practice with bare feet to allow the nadis to discharge to Earth. Try tying a cotton turban around your head to massage the cranial bones and focus your energy. If your hair is long you may practice the oldest technique to stimulate the Kundalini energy by winding the hair into a Rishi knot on top of your head.

Do not eat anything heavy for three hours before your practice, as this diverts prana to the digestive system. A light snack such as a piece of fruit is sufficient to sustain you. Drink plenty of fresh water. Humans are 75% water and high-frequency energetic practice requires water to balance the metabolic transformation engendered.

Choose a suitable surface to practice on. A sheepskin is ideal as it insulates your energy from the Earth and keeps the spine warm. A rug, thick blanket, or a standard yoga mat will all suffice, but natural materials are preferable. You will need a shawl or meditation blanket to cover yourself during deep relaxation and to wrap around your shoulders during meditation.

Ensure that your environment is as clean, clear, and uplifting as possible, to reflect your inner journey. You may find it helpful to set an altar as a focus, with a picture of a saint, a deity, an inspirational natural phenomenon, or a great teacher.

Yoga practice is beneficial at any time, but dawn and dusk are the most magical times. The sages of the East call the hours before the dawn the "amrit vela" or the "time of nectar", when the ether prevails and we are most conscious of higher frequencies.

The following are established practices to ensure your safety and enhance your experience of Kundalini Yoga.

• *Always tune in to the sacred space by chanting the Adi Mantra (see pp.53, 122).*
• *Always warm up the physical body before doing a Kundalini Yoga set or meditation.*

In the absence of other instruction:
• *All breathing is through the nose and is long, slow, and deep.*
• *Jalandhara Bandh, the Neck Lock (see p.135), should be applied at all times.*
• *The eyes should be closed with your internal focus at the Third Eye.*
• *Apply Mul Bandh, the Root Lock (see p.134) at the end of each asana and before you relax out of the posture. Inhale deeply, exhale, and apply the lock. Repeat twice more, making a total of three times.*
• *Relax with a straight spine for a minute or two between exercises to assimilate the effects of the sequence.*

1. TUNE IN

Kundalini Yoga is a self-initiatory practice; nobody else does it for you. You begin by consciously connecting to your Higher Self.

2. WARM UP

It is essential to warm up your body before any physical exercise. To prepare for your Kundalini Yoga set you could do some gentle stretches and limber-ups that are appropriate for you, or you could choose from the following warm-up exercises.

Sit comfortably in Lotus Pose (see p.131) or Easy Pose (see p.130) and apply Jalandhara Bandh, or Neck Lock (see p.135). Place your hands in Prayer Pose (see p.126). Chant the Adi Mantra once per breath, three times (see also p.122). After the third repetition breathe in and, keeping your palms together, raise your hands above your crown. Exhale and open your arms in an arc to the sides, feeling that you are opening to your Higher Self. Let your hands reach the Earth and then rest them, palms up, on your knees, straighten your spine and relax your breath, breathing long and deep.

Spinal Flex 1

Sit in Easy Pose (see p.130), holding the ankles lightly. As you inhale, flex the spine forwards, pushing your sternum forwards and up, tilting the pelvis and opening your Heart Center. On the exhale, tilt your pelvis backwards and flex your spine backwards as the lungs deflate. Your head remains level and your shoulders remain above your hips, so you are flexing the spine, not rocking back and forth.

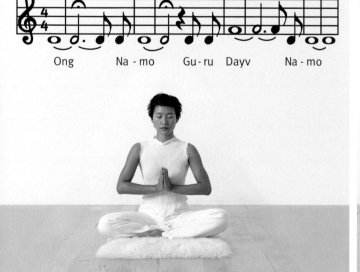

Ong   Na-mo   Gu-ru   Dayv   Na-mo

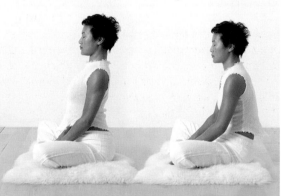

Spinal Flex 2

This exercise is identical to the last, except that your hands grasp your knees, palms-down and your arms are straight, ideally with elbows locked. The effect is to move the point of maximum flex up the spine.

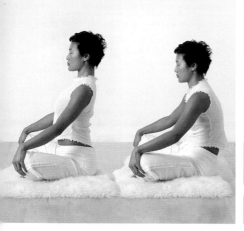

Spinal Flex 3

Sit on your heels in Rock Pose (see p.132), hands palms-down on your thighs. Flex your spine as before. The point of maximum flex is moved down your spine.

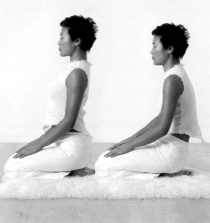

Spinal Twist

Sit in Easy Pose (see p.130), eyes closed, and grasp your right shoulder with your right hand and your left shoulder with your left. Your upper arms are at shoulder level. Breathe in as you twist your spine to the left and out as you twist to the right.

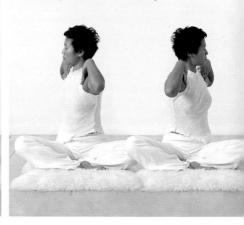

In most of these warm-up exercises, the eyes are closed and your focus is at the Third Eye. You may link your breath to a mantra by projecting "Sat" on the inhale and "Nam" on the exhale. Try to maintain each warm-up for three minutes, beginning with a slow and deliberate rhythm as you coordinate the elements of the practice for the first two minutes. Then accelerate to a comfortable but dynamic speed for the last minute.

Leg and Torso Stretch

Spread straight legs wide, knees on the ground. Hold your right toe with your right hand as you breathe out, bending your right side towards your right leg (if you cannot reach, hold your ankle or calf, or a belt around the foot). Bend your right elbow as much as you can. Gaze towards your left toe. Your left arm stretches towards your right foot. As you breathe in stretch as far as you can, still holding your toe. Continue for 2 minutes and swap legs.

Butterfly

Bring the soles of your feet together as near the perineum as possible. Clasping your feet, begin to raise your knees as you breathe in and relax them as near to the ground as possible as you breathe out.

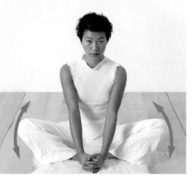

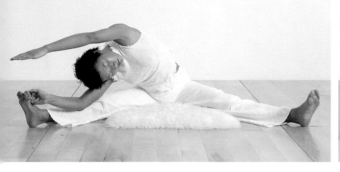

Leg Stretch

Sit with your right leg extended and bring your left ankle into the perineum, foot against your right thigh. Take your right big toe (or as far as you can reach) with both hands and bend your elbows, bringing your nose towards the knees and keeping your spine as straight as possible. Hold and begin Breath of Fire (see p.120) for thirty seconds. Change legs and repeat. Build up to 3 minutes.

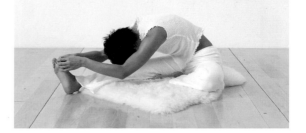

Ego Eradicator

Sit in Easy Pose (see p.130) and curl your fingers so the tips touch the pads. Your thumbs are at right-angles. Raise your arms to the sides at 60 degrees above the horizontal and do Breath of Fire (see p.120) for 3 minutes.

Breathe in and slowly bring your thumbs together above your head. Breathe out and stretch your arms down in an arc either side of the body, sweeping the auric space clean. Straighten your spine, relax the breath, and feel great.

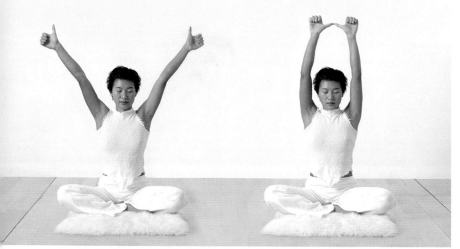

3. THE KUNDALINI YOGA KRIYA

Now you are ready to practice your chosen Kundalini Yoga kriya. Sit with a straight spine. Focus on the breath, breathing long and deep. Relax your mind and body in preparation for your chosen kriya.

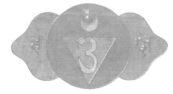

If you have not selected a kriya yet read the chakra charts on pages 35–41, complete the questionnaire on pages 43–9 and then select from the chakra kriyas on pages 64–105.

If you do not want to choose a kriya yet turn to page 61 and do Sat Kriya instead.

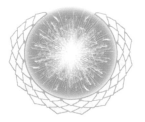

4. DEEP RELAXATION

After completing the kriya, lie in Corpse Pose (see p.129). You can cover yourself with your meditation blanket if you wish. Let your body soak into the Earth and your consciousness float free. You may relax in silence, to music, or a mantra (see p.121). Relax for 11 minutes before starting the Wake-Up Sequence.

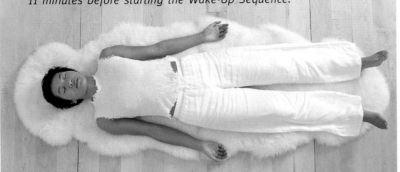

5. WAKE-UP SEQUENCE

• *Become conscious of your breath. Breathe long, slow, deep.*
• *Become conscious of the tips of your fingers and toes. Begin to flex them.*
• *Make little circles with your wrists and ankles; one way then the other.*

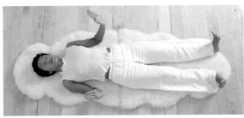

Cat Stretch

• *Stretch your arms above your head then out to the sides and breathe in, bending your right knee to your chest. Breathe out and twist your right leg and hip over your left, keeping shoulderblades on the ground. Breathe in and twist back, breathe out and lower the leg. Swap legs and repeat.*

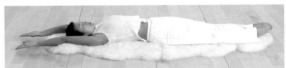

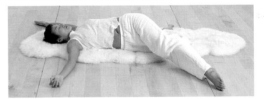

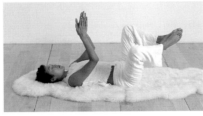

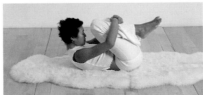

• *Rub your soles and palms together.*
• *Hug your knees to your chest and rock from side to side.*
• *Rock along the length of your spine. (Take care that you round your spine and that you are lying on a soft surface.)*

6. THE KUNDALINI YOGA MEDITATION

Now you are ready to practice your chosen Kundalini Yoga meditation.

Come into your chosen sitting posture. Focus on the breath, breathing long and deep. Relax the mind and body in preparation for your chosen meditation. Choose your meditation by deciding which of your yogic bodies you are going to work on, see pp.17–31. If you have not yet chosen a meditation turn to page 62 and do Kirtan Kriya Meditation instead.

7. COMPLETION

i *After completing your meditation, seal your practice by sitting in Prayer Pose (see p.126) in a state of heart-centered neutrality and singing.*

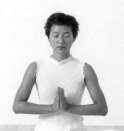

"Why do we meditate? These thoughts, which the subconscious, the id, releases; some we deal with some we don't deal with. Those we don't deal with go into the subconscious. Meditation is nothing but a self-invoked dream. The proper translation of meditation is, 'Self-Invoked Hypnotic Dream in which you Clean Your Subconscious'.

When somebody says, 'I had a dream of this, I had a dream of that,' actually what you are dreaming comes from your subconscious. And then you have day-dreaming, you have night-dreaming, you have nightmares. That is when the subconscious starts unloading into the unconsciousness. If you meditate, you are not doing anybody any favour, and you are not going to grow wings from your armpits. It will only help you to be a self-controlled person. It will only mean people will respect you, trust you and like you. You will not have a split personality, and your words will mean exactly what you are saying. That's all. It's no big miracle. If you don't meditate you won't be true to yourself."

Yogi Bhajan, The Master's Touch, 21st April 1997

This final mantra affirms your identity as living in truth and is chanted once per breath in either the long form, where the Sat is 8 times longer than the Nam (see below) or in the longest form, where the Sat is 35 times longer than the Nam. The sound "Sat" rises from the base of the spine to the center of the head; the sound "Nam" radiates out to Infinity; the in-breath completes the cycle, returning your awareness to the physical body upon the Earth.

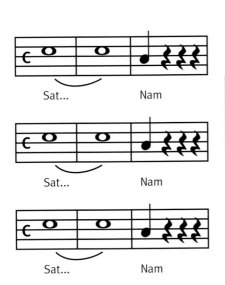

Sat...   Nam

Sat...   Nam

Sat...   Nam

ii *Breathe in deeply. Keeping the hands in Prayer Pose raise them high.*

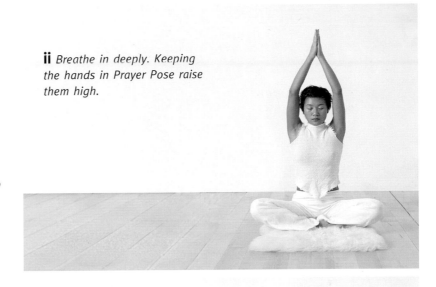

Breathe out and be consciously aware of the energy moving down through the chakras as you bring your hands down above the crown, before the Third Eye, the throat, and the heart.

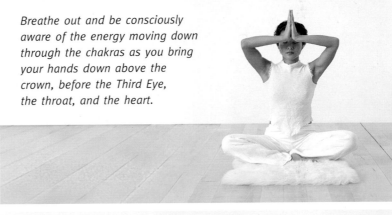

Bend forwards and bow as you separate the hands and bring the palms on to the ground. Sat Nam.

Part 3

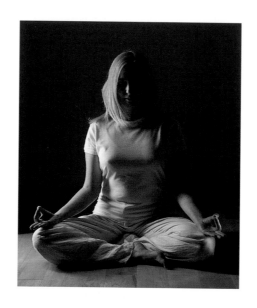

the kriyas and meditations

A Kriya and Meditation for Everyone for Every Day

Sat Kriya

• *Sit in Rock Pose (see p.132).
Clasp your hands together, extending and pressing your index fingers
together. For women, the left thumb
is on top of the right; for men, vice
versa. Stretch your arms vertically,
elbows hugging your ears.*
• *Begin to chant "Sat Nam" at 8
repetitions per 10 seconds. As you
chant "Sat" pull your navel in and
up. As you chant "Nam" relax and
release. Continue for 3 minutes.*
• *To finish, breathe in, and apply
Maha Bandh (see p.135). Contract
your buttocks and genital muscles,
squeezing the energy up your spine,
pulling in your navel and lifting
your diaphragm. Tucking in your
chin and extending your neck, turn
your eyes up to look out of your
crown. Mentally feel the flow of
subtle energy.*
• *Now relax for at least 6 minutes.*

*Increase your practice until you can
sustain 31 minutes and relax for
twice as long as your practice.*

Sat Kriya and Kirtan Kriya
Meditation *(see next page)*
are suitable for everyone, every
day. Once you are familiar with
the format for your Kundalini
Yoga experience replace them
with your own selection.

Yogi Bhajan comments:
*Sat Kriya is a key kriya of Kundalini
Yoga and should be practiced daily
for at least 3 minutes. Relax for
6 minutes afterwards. Sat Kriya
strengthens the sexual system and
stimulates energy flow. It eases
sexual phobias, and channels sexual
energy into other creative areas.
The internal organs benefit from its
rhythmic massage. Sat Kriya directly
stimulates the Kundalini energy, so
it must be practiced with "Sat Nam".
Respect the power of the technique.
It is a kriya that works on all levels
of your being, known and unknown.*

Kirtan Kriya Meditation

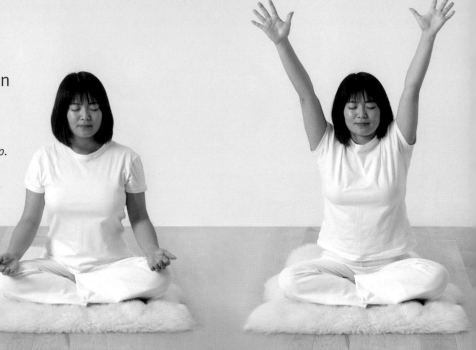

Sit in Easy Pose (see p.130), hands resting on knees, palms up. Close your eyes and focus in the center of the head. As you chant, experience the mantra entering through the crown and exiting through the Third Eye, making a right-angle, visualizing the Golden Cord (see p.136) connecting the pineal and pituitary glands.

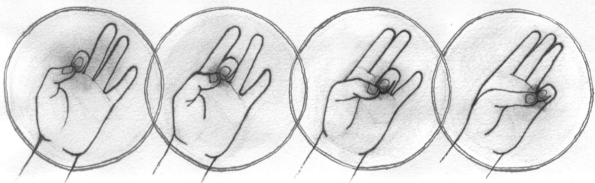

- *Chant "Sa" and press the index fingertip to the thumb (Gyan Mudra)*

- *Chant "Ta" and press middle fingertip to the thumb (Shuni Mudra).*

- *Chant "Na" and press the ring fingertip to the thumb (Surya Mudra).*

- *Chant "Ma" and press the little fingertip to the thumb (Bhuddhi Mudra).*

- *Chant aloud for 5 minutes using the notes A G F G (see below).*
- *Chant in a whisper for 5 minutes.*
- *Chant silently for 11 minutes.*
- *Chant in a whisper for 5 minutes.*
- *Chant aloud for 5 minutes, as before.*

To finish, breathe in. Breathe out. Breathe in and stretch your arms as high as possible. Breathe out and continue to stretch. Breathe in and relax the arms down, and relax.

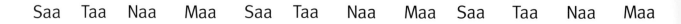

Saa   Taa   Naa   Maa   Saa   Taa   Naa   Maa   Saa   Taa   Naa   Maa

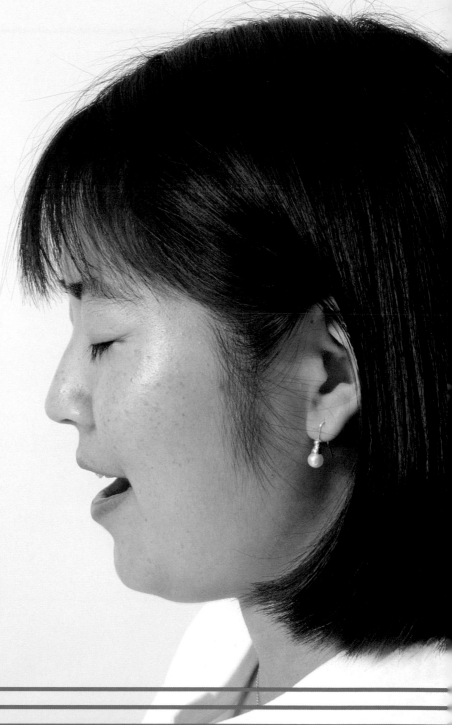

Yogi Bhajan comments:
*All meditation begins and ends
with Sa Ta Na Ma.
Sa sound of Infinity, Ta sound of life,
Na sound of conquering death,
Ma sound of resurrection.
All that is contained in Christ
Consciousness is hidden in the four
folds of this word into the fifth of
Infinity. May the consciousness
become higher and higher and higher,
of the highest. May we sacrifice the
ego to receive, and resurrect our own
Self into the domain of Light to the
Grace of God to merge in God itself.
Sat Nam.*

*In the beginning all was one and
the sound of all was a never-ending
Aaaaa. The other four primal sounds,
S T N M, found expression through
the fifth and created SaTaNaMa, a
wave form that anticipates the cycle
of creation; the snake eating its tail;
life, death, and rebirth into the
Infinity from which life sprang
and which is represented in this
meditation by a musical wave
form (see below).
We chant in the three languages
of consciousness, representing the
three ages of the great cycle:*
1 *The everyday human voice of the
Base Metal Age we are living through.*
2 *The whisper of lovers in the dark
who remember the Silver Age of myth
and legend.*
3 *The silence of the Divine; the
Golden Age that was and will be
when All are One.*

Saa   Taa   Naa   Maa   Saa   Taa   Naa   Maa   Saa   Taa   Naa   Maa

First Chakra
MULADHARA

1a   Kriya for the First Chakra

Originally taught by Yogi Bhajan as KRIYA FOR LOWER SPINE AND ELIMINATION

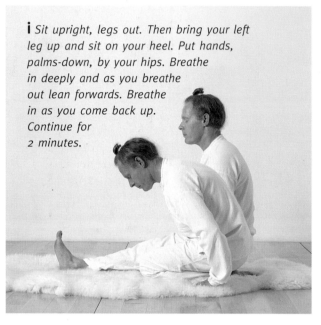

i *Sit upright, legs out. Then bring your left leg up and sit on your heel. Put hands, palms-down, by your hips. Breathe in deeply and as you breathe out lean forwards. Breathe in as you come back up. Continue for 2 minutes.*

ii *Now do the same as in* **i***, but with both legs out. Continue for 2 minutes.*

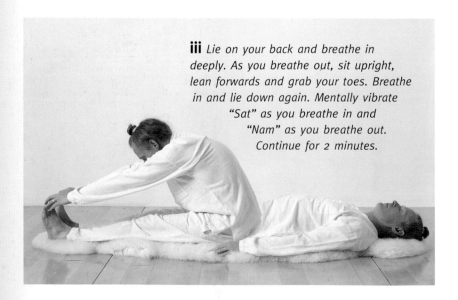

iii *Lie on your back and breathe in deeply. As you breathe out, sit upright, lean forwards and grab your toes. Breathe in and lie down again. Mentally vibrate "Sat" as you breathe in and "Nam" as you breathe out. Continue for 2 minutes.*

PLOUGH POSE Beginner's variation: place a chair behind you to rest your toes on, rather than over-stretching by trying to reach the floor.

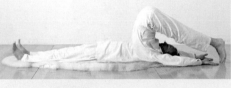

iv *Lying on your back, arms behind your head, lift your legs until your feet touch the ground. This is Plough Pose (see also p.132).*

Then allow your legs back down, sit up, and grab your toes. Carry on alternating between Plough Pose and forward-stretching, without pausing, for 2 minutes.

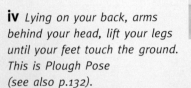

v *Lie on your back and clasp your knees. Stretch your legs out before sitting up to grab your toes. Continue for 2 minutes in a steady rhythm.*

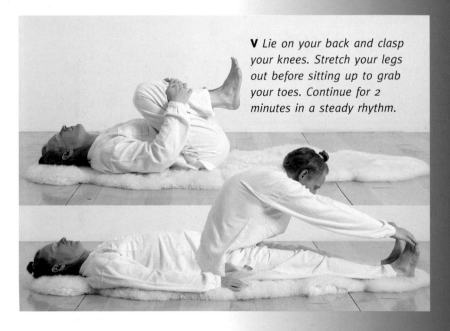

vi *With both legs extended, bend forwards to grab your toes. As you roll back on your spine, hold on to your toes until you are in Plough Pose (see p.132). Roll backwards and forwards without letting go of your toes. Continue for 2 minutes.*

Beginner's variation: Put a belt around your feet to extend your arms.

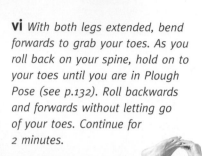

vii *Relax completely.*

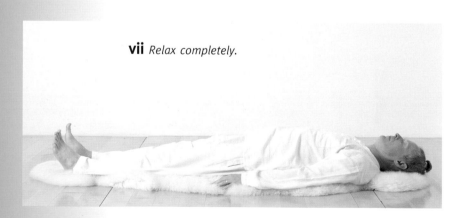

Yogi Bhajan comments:
The First, Second, and Third Chakras, associated with the rectum, sex organs, and Navel Point are thoroughly exercised, giving flexibility to the spine and improving digestion and elimination.

1b   Kriya for the First Chakra

Originally taught by Yogi Bhajan as WORKING ON THE LOWER SPINE April 24th 1985

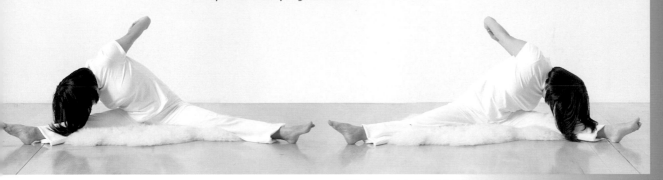

i *Sitting, spread your legs wide and clasp your hands behind you in Venus Lock (see p.127). Bend to the left and touch your nose to your left knee as you lift your arms high. Then bend to the right and touch your nose to the right knee. Chant "Har" as you bend down and "Haray" as you come up. Continue for 5 minutes.*

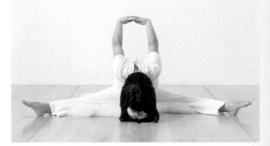

ii *Continue as in **i**, but now additionally bend forwards to the center. Bend to the left and touch the nose to the left knee as you lift your arms high. Then bend to the center, lifting your arms. Then bend to the right and touch your nose to your knee. Chant "Har" as you bend down and "Haray" as you come up. Continue for 2 minutes.*

iii *Remain sitting, legs spread, hands locked in front, and raise your arms. Now keep your arms straight as you twist your torso rapidly left and right. Continue for 2 minutes.*
• Loosens up the lower rib cage and lungs.

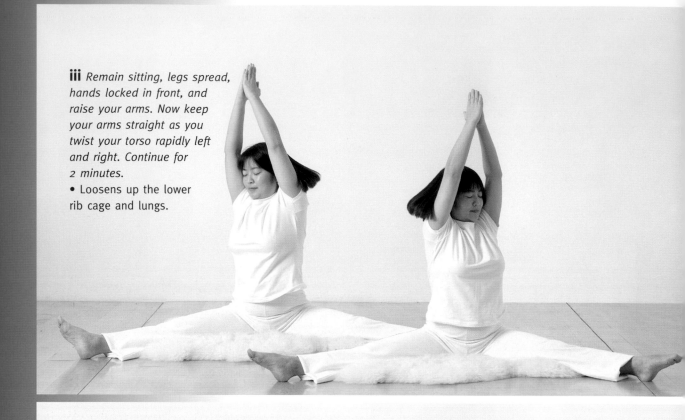

iv *Remain sitting with your legs wide; bend your elbows, clasp your hands in front, and twist vigorously left and right for 2 minutes.*
• Use anger to fuel this movement; it is not gentle, it has to be wild.

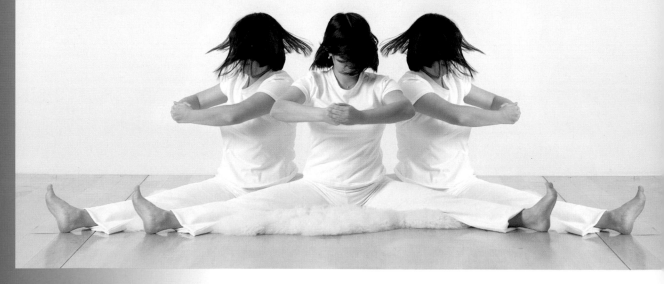

V *With legs still spread wide, lie on your back and rest your clasped hands on your navel. Stick the tip of your tongue out and roll the sides up. Begin Breath of Fire (see p.120). Keeping your legs still and your spine as straight as you can, sit up and lie back down. Maintain a steady rhythm and continue for 5 minutes.*

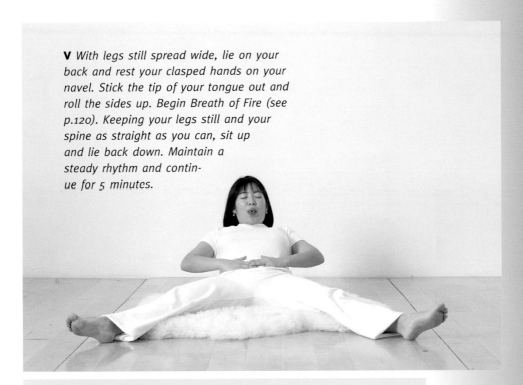

vi *Squat in Frog Pose (see p.130). With eyes closed, place your hands on the ground and meditate at Third Eye. Breathe in and straighten your legs, raising your buttocks, hands on the ground. Heels should remain off the ground. Breathe out and return to the squat. Pull your Navel Point sharply in, twice, breath held out. One repetition of the cycle will take 2½ seconds. Continue for 5 minutes.*
• *Tunes all the organs of the body.*

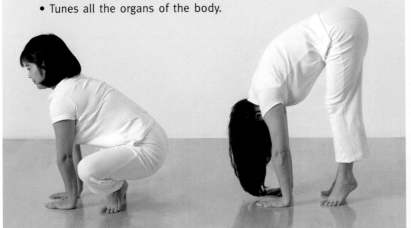

vi *In Easy Pose (see p.130), meditate at the Third Eye for 2 minutes.*

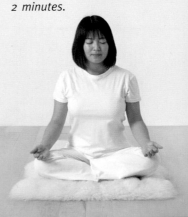

Second Chakra
SVADHISTHANA

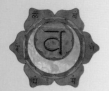

2a Kriya for the Second Chakra

Originally taught by Yogi Bhajan as KRIYA FOR PELVIC BALANCE

> **Important:**
> This is a strenuous set of exercises, and it is vital to do a short set of warm-up exercises first (see pp.53–7), to warm and flex the spine. If you are a beginner approach these exercises slowly and carefully.

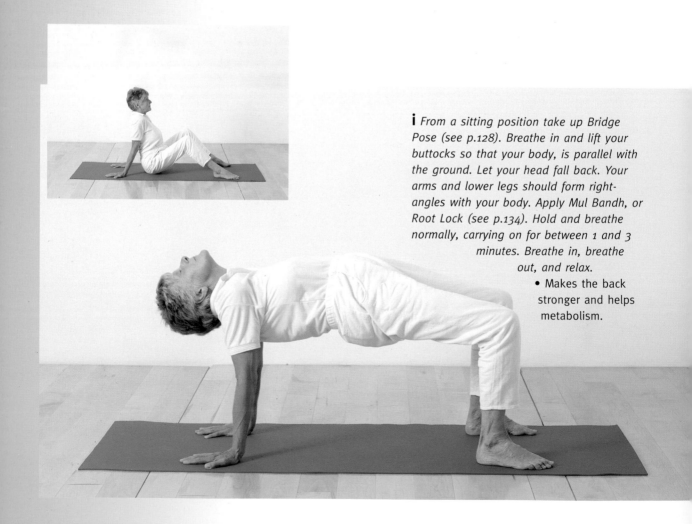

i *From a sitting position take up Bridge Pose (see p.128). Breathe in and lift your buttocks so that your body, is parallel with the ground. Let your head fall back. Your arms and lower legs should form right-angles with your body. Apply Mul Bandh, or Root Lock (see p.134). Hold and breathe normally, carrying on for between 1 and 3 minutes. Breathe in, breathe out, and relax.*

• Makes the back stronger and helps metabolism.

ii *Prepare as shown and take up Wheel Pose (see p.133). Breathe in and raise your buttocks, so that your body forms a single bridge. Begin Breath of Fire (see p.120). Continue for 1 to 3 minutes. Breathe in, let yourself down, and relax.*
• Helps to strengthen the lower back, causing energy flow through the spine, and aiding metabolism.

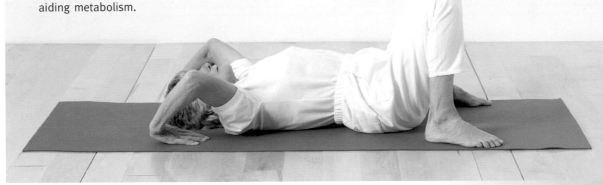

iii *Lie on your front, hands in Venus Lock (see p.127) behind. Breathe in and lift your legs and arms, keeping knees and elbows as straight as possible. Begin Breath of Fire (see p.120) and continue for 1 to 3 minutes. Breathe in, breathe out, and relax.*
• Helps digestion and strengthens the abdominals.

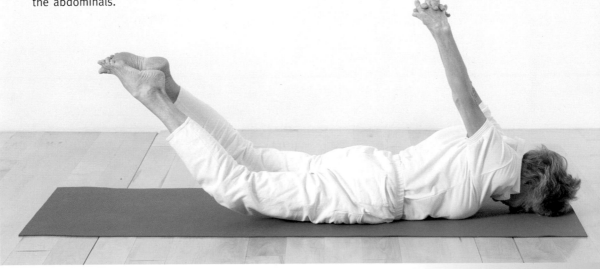

iv *With feet wide apart, lift your arms, palms together. Breathe in. Breathe out, bending at the waist, and touch your left foot with your fingertips. Breathe in as you come up and then out, bending and touching your right foot. Continue rhythmically, with powerful breathing, for 1 to 3 minutes. Then inhale into the upright position. Breathe out and relax.*
• Balances the movement of the pelvis and coordinates muscle groups on opposite sides of the body.

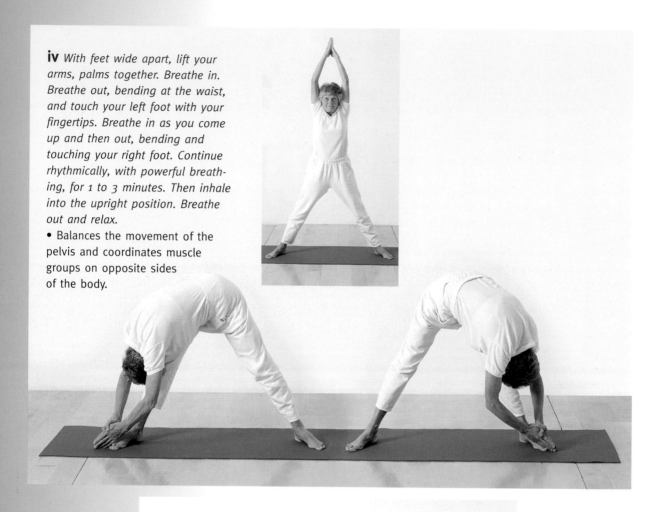

v *Assume Kundalini Lotus (see p.131). Open your legs wide and begin Breath of Fire (see p.120). Continue for 1 to 3 minutes. Breathe in and out and relax.*
• Helps channel sexual energy and maintain potency.

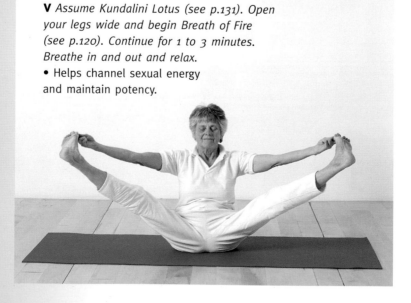

vi *Move into Cow Pose (see p.129).*
Breathe in, lifting your head up and back
and lifting your right leg high, knee as
straight as possible. Breathe out; bring
your chin to your chest and draw your right
knee to your head. Then breathe in and
return to the original position. Continue
rhythmically, with powerful breathing, for 1
to 3 minutes. Then breathe in. Breathe out.
Repeat for the other side. Continue for 1 to
3 minutes. Then breathe in. Breathe out
and relax.
• Balances the leg and abdominals and
helps maintain sexual potency.

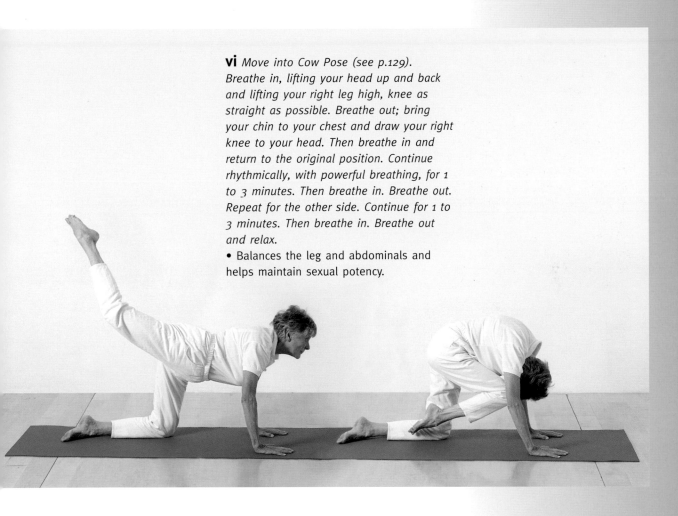

vii *Relax deeply.*

Yogi Bhajan comments:
To walk with grace and strength is to feel connected to the world and
ready to act. This is not only a matter of mindset but also of physical
balance. When the pelvis and its muscles are out of balance, many
systems begin to show stress. Exhaustion, low endurance, and lower
back pain are common symptoms. This kriya is helpful for staying ener-
getic and balanced. It helps to maintain potency if practiced regularly.

2b   Kriya for the Second Chakra

Originally taught by Yogi Bhajan as SEXUALITY AND SPIRITUALITY on April 16th 1986

This kriya could not be verified by KRI and therefore is not certified as accurate. (See website address p.143.)

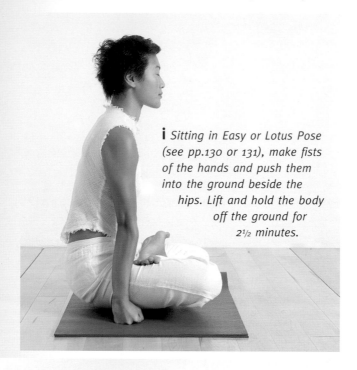

i *Sitting in Easy or Lotus Pose (see pp.130 or 131), make fists of the hands and push them into the ground beside the hips. Lift and hold the body off the ground for 2½ minutes.*

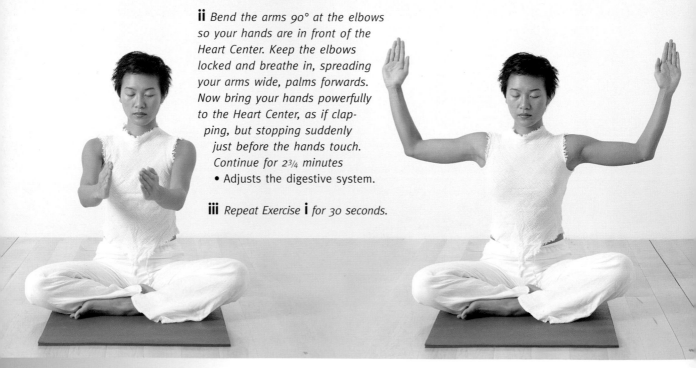

ii *Bend the arms 90° at the elbows so your hands are in front of the Heart Center. Keep the elbows locked and breathe in, spreading your arms wide, palms forwards. Now bring your hands powerfully to the Heart Center, as if clapping, but stopping suddenly just before the hands touch. Continue for 2¾ minutes*
• *Adjusts the digestive system.*

iii *Repeat Exercise i for 30 seconds.*

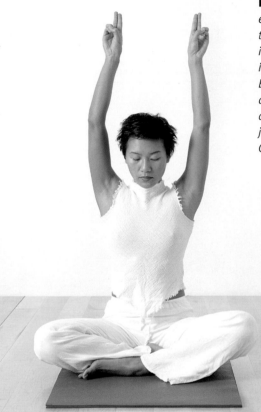

iv *Bend the ring and little finger of each hand to the palm and place the thumb on top. Extend your index and middle fingers. Breathe in as you raise your arms high. Breathe out as you bring your arms down to Earth as powerfully as you can, stopping suddenly just before touching the ground. Continue for 1½ minutes.*

v *With eyes closed, focus on the Third Eye. Make fists of your hands, place them in front of your Heart Center, and wind them rapidly around each other. Continue for 4½ minutes.*

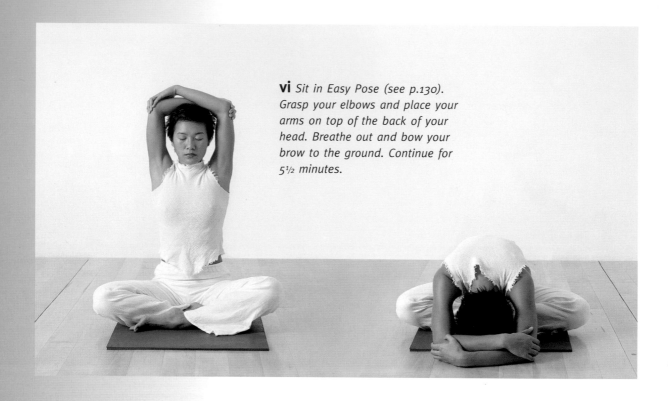

vi *Sit in Easy Pose (see p.130). Grasp your elbows and place your arms on top of the back of your head. Breathe out and bow your brow to the ground. Continue for 5½ minutes.*

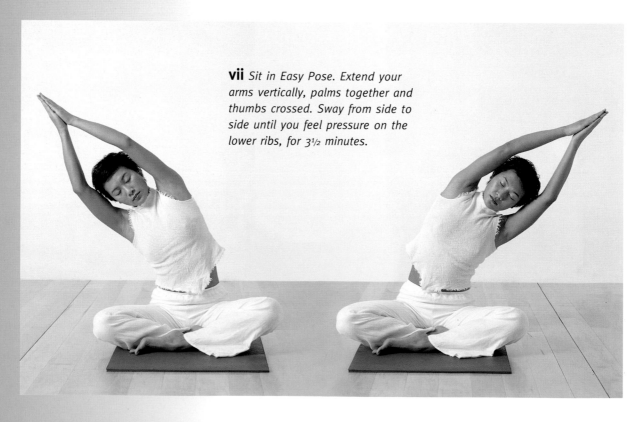

vii *Sit in Easy Pose. Extend your arms vertically, palms together and thumbs crossed. Sway from side to side until you feel pressure on the lower ribs, for 3½ minutes.*

viii *Lie on your back. Clasp your hands behind your neck in Venus Lock (see p.127). Push your pelvis rapidly up and down (15–22 cm/ 6–9 in), keeping your heels and shoulders on the ground. Point your toes. Continue for 5 minutes.*
• Creates a special Pranayam.

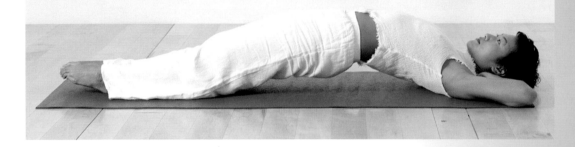

ix *Relax in Corpse Pose (see p.129) for 3½ minutes.*

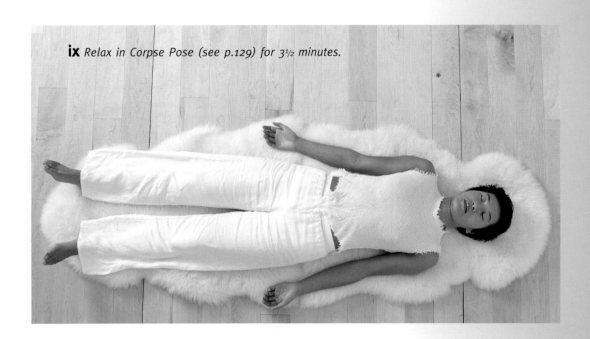

Third Chakra
MANIPURA

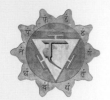

3a   Kriya for the Third Chakra

Originally taught by Yogi Bhajan as BEGINNERS' CLEANSING SET

i *Put hands in Venus Lock (see p.127) at the back of your neck. Begin Breath of Fire (see p.120) for 90 seconds, breathe in, and hold for 20 seconds. Repeat Breath of Fire, breathe in, and hold for 30 seconds. Relax the breath. Breathe in deeply, lifting both legs 30 cm (12 in). Hold for 15 seconds, breathe out, breathe in, and relax.*

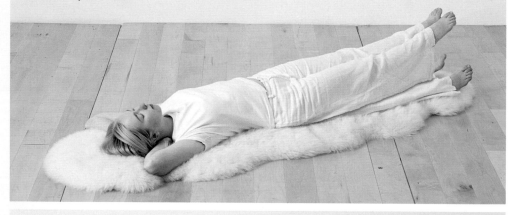

ii *Spread your legs wide. Begin Breath of Fire (see p.120) for 1 minute. Breathe in, raising your legs 90 cm (3 ft) and hold for 5 seconds. Relax your legs. Repeat 3 times, doing Breath of Fire for 1 minute each time. Repeat Breath of Fire once more then breathe in, raising your legs 30 cm (12 in). Hold as long as you feel you can.*
• Stimulates the sex energy channels in the upper thighs.

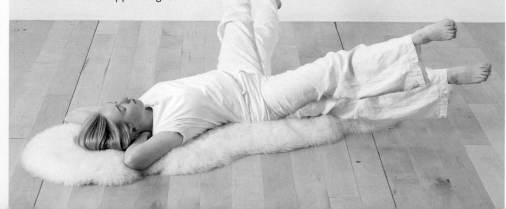

iii *Lie in Stretch Pose (see p.132) and lift your heels 15 cm (6 in). Lift your head and shoulders 15 cm (6 in) and look towards your toes. Begin Breath of Fire (see p.120) and continue for 3 minutes. Breathe in and relax.*

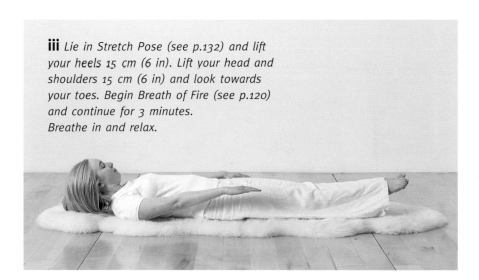

iv *Sit upright, legs extended. Put your left foot on your right thigh. Keep your hands parallel to the ground, either side of your extended foot. Breathe in, breathe out, and reach past your toes. Breathe in deeply and sit up, leaning back to 30 degrees. Breathe out. Repeat 25 times and swap legs.*

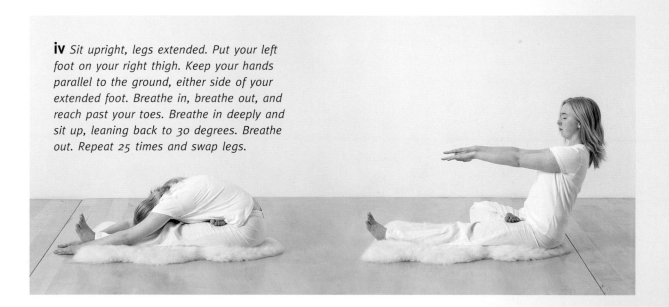

v *Sit upright and lean back 30 degrees. Let your arms support your upper body. Drop your head back and gaze at a chosen spot without blinking. Begin Breath of Fire (see p.120) for 2 minutes. Breathe in and lift both feet 30 cm (12 in), hold your gaze. Hold for 15 to 20 seconds; breathe out, down. Repeat Breath of Fire for 1 minute. Breathe in, raising both feet 30 cm (12 in). Hold for 15 seconds. Breathe out and relax totally on your back.*

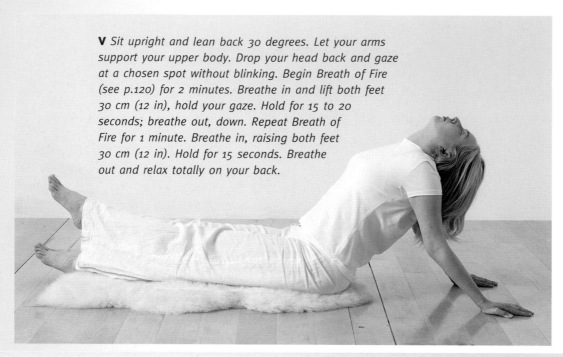

vi *On your back, eyes closed, breathe in deeply and completely. Lift your hands, with fingers stretched. Make tight fists and slowly bring them to your chest. Tense your arms, so that your fists shake. Relax your breath. Repeat, breath held in, before relaxing deeply and completely for 5 minutes.*

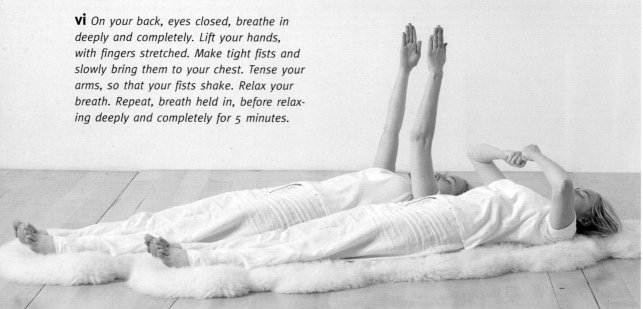

Yogi Bhajan comments:
*Step **i** stimulates the Navel Point energy and blood circulation into the lungs. Step **ii** adds the creative power of sexual energy. Step **iii** re-stimulates the Navel Point. Step **iv** adjusts the chemical balance in the blood and helps the lower back and waistline. Step **v** moves the energy into the brain and eyes. Step **vi** removes residual tension and allows you to relax.*

3b Kriya for the Third Chakra

Originally taught by Yogi Bhajan as NABHI KRIYA FOR PRANA-APANA

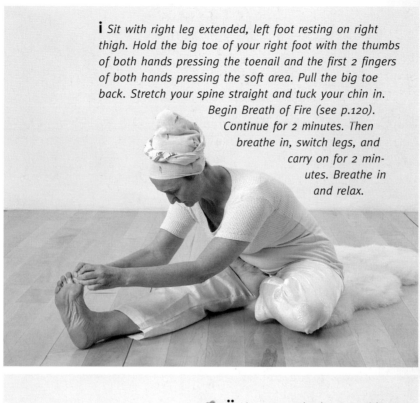

i *Sit with right leg extended, left foot resting on right thigh. Hold the big toe of your right foot with the thumbs of both hands pressing the toenail and the first 2 fingers of both hands pressing the soft area. Pull the big toe back. Stretch your spine straight and tuck your chin in. Begin Breath of Fire (see p.120). Continue for 2 minutes. Then breathe in, switch legs, and carry on for 2 minutes. Breathe in and relax.*

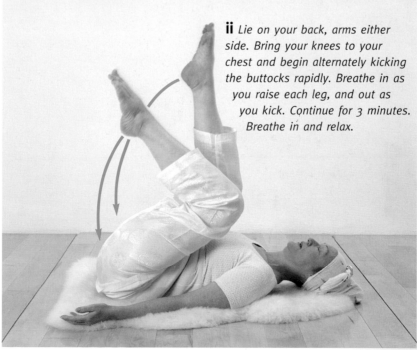

ii *Lie on your back, arms either side. Bring your knees to your chest and begin alternately kicking the buttocks rapidly. Breathe in as you raise each leg, and out as you kick. Continue for 3 minutes. Breathe in and relax.*

iii *Lift your legs 45 cm (18 in). Breathe in and draw your left knee to your chest. Breathe out as you stretch out your left leg and, at the same time, draw your right knee to your chest, keeping the lower leg parallel with the floor. Continue, combined with deep, strong breathing, for 3 minutes. Breathe in and stretch out both legs. Breathe out and relax.*

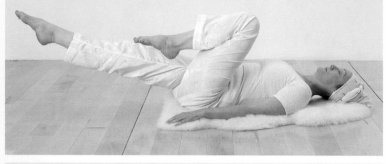

iv *On your front, raise yourself on your hands until the elbows lock. Your body forms a straight line. Begin Breath of Fire (see p.120) and carry on for 3 minutes. Breathe in and hold, then breathe out. Breathe in. Then breathe out completely and hold it out briefly. Breathe in and relax.*

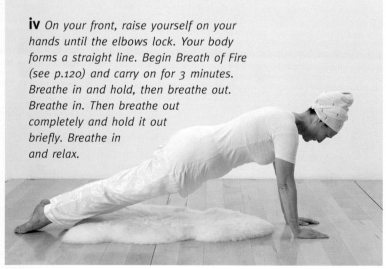

v *Take up Stretch Pose (see p.132). Lift your head and shoulders 15 cm (6 in) and gaze towards your toes, arms outstretched. Breathe in and hold before breathing out. Breathe in. Breathe out completely and apply Mul Bandh, or Root Lock (see p.134). Breathe in and relax.*

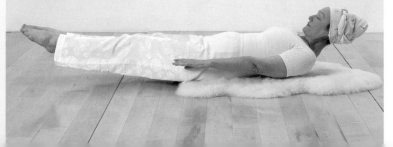

vi *Assume Easy Pose (see p.130). Spread your arms to form an angle of 60 degrees. Tense the fingers.*

Take several long, deep breaths, and make tight fists, bringing them slowly to your chest, and then breathing out forcefully. Repeat 2 to 3 times.

Spreading the arms again, tense the fingers and breathe long and deep. Bring your hands 10 cm (4 in) apart in front. Gazing at the space between the palms, feel energy flowing between them. Continue long, deep breathing for 1 to 2 minutes.

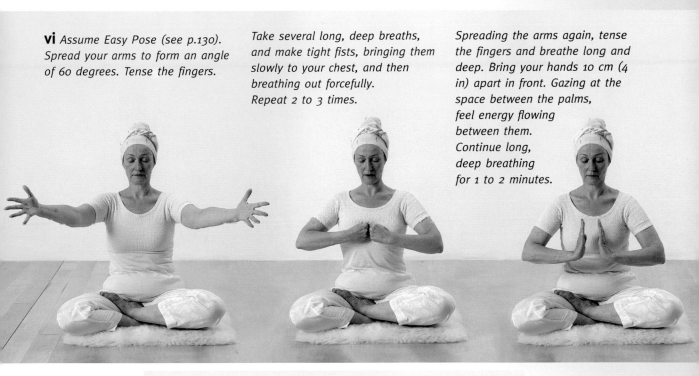

Then bring palms together at your chest. Meditate at the Third Eye for 1 minute. Then, bending from the waist, finally bring your forehead and palms flat to the floor (not shown). Relax in this position for 1 to 2 minutes.

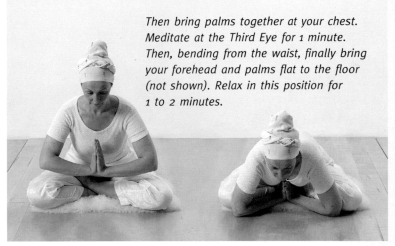

vii *Sit up and meditate for 11 minutes.*

viii *Relax in Corpse Pose (see p.129) for 11 minutes.*

Yogi Bhajan comments:
*This kriya is good for strength, digestion, abdominal toning, mild depression, and for developing the healing flow of prana through the hands. Exercise **i** opens the lungs, balances the aura, and stimulates the pituitary. Exercises **ii** and **iii** aid digestion. Exercise **iv** strengthens the lower back and stimulates the brain. Exercise **v** balances the Third Chakra, sets the Navel Point, and aids digestion. Exercise **vi** brings mental and physical focus to the hands and opens the Heart Center.*

Fourth Chakra
ANAHATA

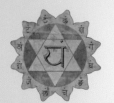

4a   Kriya for the Fourth Chakra

Originally taught by Yogi Bhajan as

EXERCISE TO STRENGTHEN THE NERVOUS SYSTEM AND OPEN THE HEART

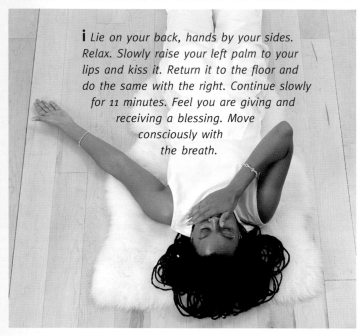

i *Lie on your back, hands by your sides. Relax. Slowly raise your left palm to your lips and kiss it. Return it to the floor and do the same with the right. Continue slowly for 11 minutes. Feel you are giving and receiving a blessing. Move consciously with the breath.*

ii *With eyes closed, bend your knees to your chest, tucking your hands in behind your knees. Hold tightly and bring your legs over the head, parallel to the ground. Slowly bend your knees and return to the starting position. Continue steadily for 5 minutes.*

iii *Relax.*

Yogi Bhajan comments:
Makes you feel good and makes deep breathing automatic. Automatic pranayama increases circulation all over the body. 15 minutes each day can make you feel young, happy, beautiful, and healthy.

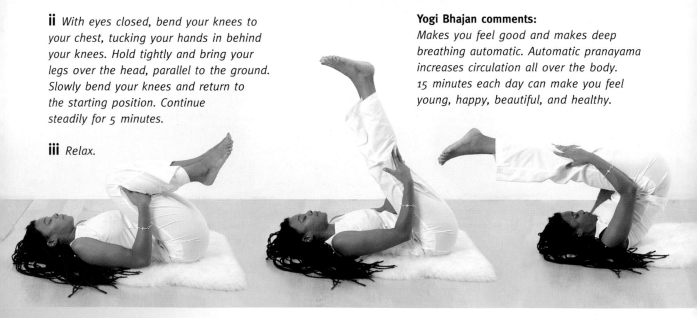

4b   Kriya for the Fourth Chakra

Originally taught by Yogi Bhajan as OPPORTUNITY AND GREEN ENERGY SET

i *Sit in Rock Pose (see p.132). Breathe in and flex the upper body forwards, mentally chanting "Sat", focusing at the First Chakra. Breathe out and flex backwards, mentally chanting "Nam" and focus on the Third Chakra for 2 minutes. To finish, breathe in, apply Mul Bandh (see p.134), breathe out, apply Mul Bandh, and hold 10 seconds. Repeat 3 times.*

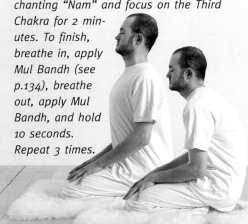

ii *Sit with your legs stretched out. Place your hands beside your hips. Push down, lifting your body (and legs) momentarily off the floor before letting it drop again. Keep your spine vertical. Continue rapidly for 2 minutes.*

iii *Squat in Crow Pose (see p.130), spine straight. Clasp your hands, index fingers straight out. Extend the arms at heart level. Look into Infinity. Maintain with Breath of Fire (see p.120) for 2 minutes. To finish, breathe in and hold as long as you can while continuing to project out from the Heart Center.*

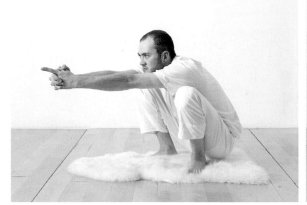

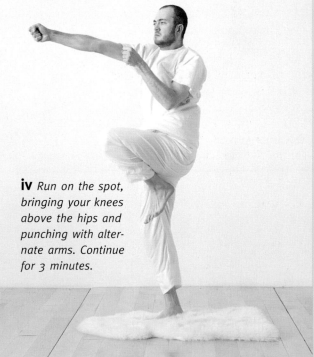

iv *Run on the spot, bringing your knees above the hips and punching with alternate arms. Continue for 3 minutes.*

v *Assume Kundalini Lotus (see p.131). Hold with Breath of Fire (see p.120) for 2 minutes. To finish, breathe in and hold while drawing energy up the spine. Breathe out and relax.*

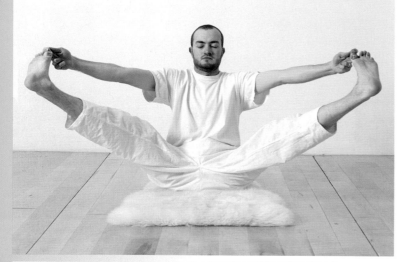

vi *Sit on your left heel, with right foot on left thigh. Cup your hands just below the navel. Pull your diaphragm up and chant "Ong So Hung" powerfully from the heart for 3 minutes.*

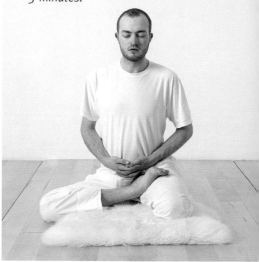

vii *Sit in Easy Pose (see p.130), eyes closed. Extend your arms, palms up. Visualize energy arching over your head, flowing in through your left palm and out the right. Continue with Breath of Fire (see p.120) for 2 minutes. To finish, breathe in and hold as long as you can, continuing to feel the flow of energy. Exhale and relax.*

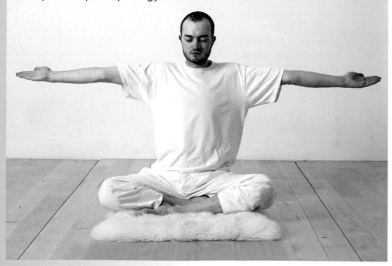

viii *Sit in Easy Pose (see p.130), placing your hands in Venus Lock (see p.127) behind your neck. Breathe in and bring your forehead to the floor, mentally chanting "Sat". Breathe out and come up, mentally chanting "Nam". Continue for 2 minutes.*

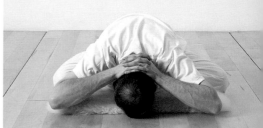

ix *Sit in Easy Pose (see p.130), arms extended. Breathe in and raise your right arm to 60 degrees, breathe out and lower to horizontal. Breathe in and raise your left arm to 60 degrees, breathe out and lower to horizontal. Continue moving rapidly for 2 minutes. To finish, bring your arms together at the brow level, breathe in, hold the breath, projecting from the Third Eye to Infinity. Breathe out and relax.*

x *Sit in Easy Pose, hands in Venus Lock (see p.127), 10 cm (4 in) above the Seventh Chakra. Look out of this chakra. Hold with Breath of Fire (see p.120) for 2 minutes. Then extend index fingers and breathe long and deep for 2 minutes. Continue, but open the hands so only finger- and thumbtips touch and hold with Breath of Fire for 2 minutes. Breathe in and hold, projecting up and out. Breathe out and relax.*

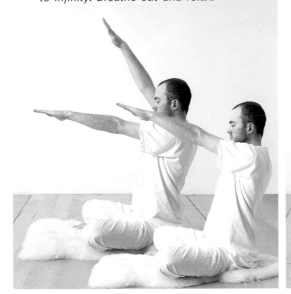

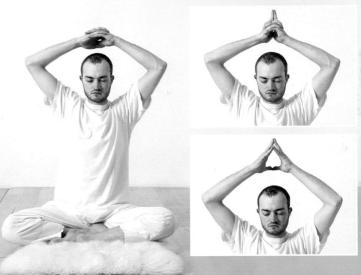

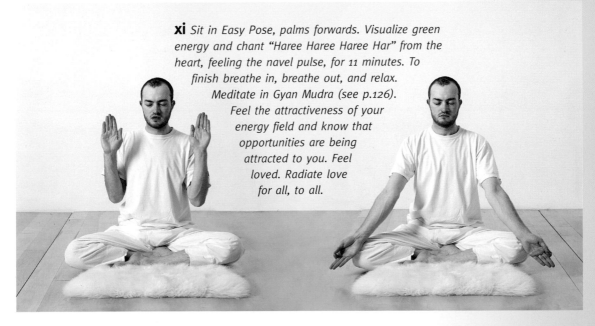

xi *Sit in Easy Pose, palms forwards. Visualize green energy and chant "Haree Haree Haree Har" from the heart, feeling the navel pulse, for 11 minutes. To finish breathe in, breathe out, and relax. Meditate in Gyan Mudra (see p.126). Feel the attractiveness of your energy field and know that opportunities are being attracted to you. Feel loved. Radiate love for all, to all.*

Fifth Chakra
VISHUDDHA

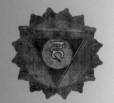

5a Kriya for the Fifth Chakra
Originally taught by Yogi Bhajan as FOR CREATIVITY

i *Sit on your heels, palms together, and lower your forehead to the ground, arms extended. Breathe in and imagine energy moving to the spine base. Hold the breath and let rainbow colours spread up your spine, from red at the base to violet at the crown. Breathe out and let the colours dissipate. Breathe in and begin again. Continue for up to 5 minutes.*

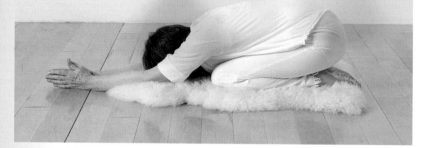

ii *Sit up, extend your legs, and lean back 30 degrees, supported by your arms, and let your head fall back. Relax. Breathe deeply for 3 minutes. Use your abdominals and chest muscles. On each out-breath imagine a beam of light shining from your forehead. On the last breath, hold, then sigh out through your nose, slowly letting yourself down on to your back to relax.*

iii *After relaxing, sit in Easy Pose (see p.130), with fingers interlaced. Breathe in deeply and chant "Ong" evenly. Make the sound last as long as possible. Pull your chin in, so that when you make the "ng" sound, you can feel vibration moving into the cranium, gently stimulating the brain. Continue for 11 minutes.*

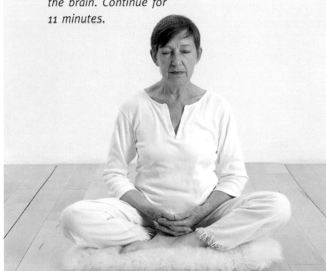

iv *Sit in Easy Pose and press your palms together at the Heart Center, thumbs in firm contact. Draw your concentration to the Heart Center for 2 minutes.*

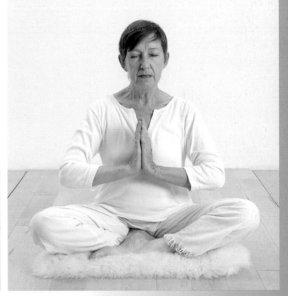

v *Rub your palms together energetically, producing heat, for 2 minutes, feeling the build-up of energy. Hold the palms 10 cm (4 in) apart, and feel the opposites of attraction and repulsion: right palm positive, left palm negative. Close your eyes and do this for 2 minutes.*

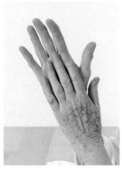
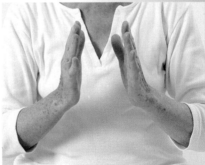

vi *Cup your hands, right palm down, left palm up, and hold 10 cm (4 in) apart, at the level of the heart. Breathe deeply and calmly, collecting breath energy between the palms and visualizing it as a sphere of glowing light. Do this for 4 minutes. Relax and smile; you are opening your heart.*

vii *With eyes closed, press your right palm to the Heart Center and press your left hand on your spine, palm out, opposite your right palm. Experience the build-up of charging polarity and begin Breath of Fire (see p.120), using the navel as a pump. After 2 minutes, breathe in, hold, and breathe out. Meditate for a few minutes, back straight, hands in your lap. Experience your own sacredness.*

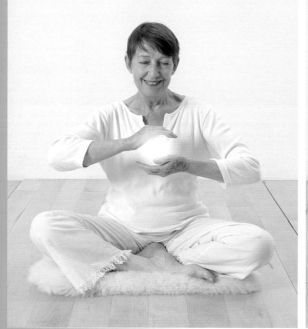

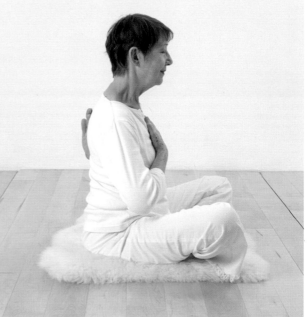

Yogi Bhajan comments:

An artist takes great care of his tools. Yet the fundamental tool, the mind, is left wandering, full of conflicting desires. It is necessary to be able to tune the mind to the basic life forces, and to be able to relax the mental processes so that spontaneous creative impulses can come through. These exercises are useful if they are done regularly, whenever you want to be creative.

5b Kriya for the Fifth Chakra

Originally taught by Yogi Bhajan as
FOR CREATIVITY

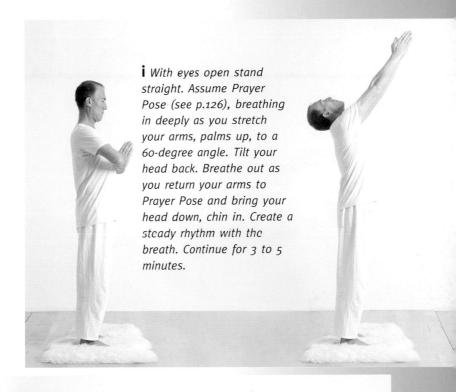

i *With eyes open stand straight. Assume Prayer Pose (see p.126), breathing in deeply as you stretch your arms, palms up, to a 60-degree angle. Tilt your head back. Breathe out as you return your arms to Prayer Pose and bring your head down, chin in. Create a steady rhythm with the breath. Continue for 3 to 5 minutes.*

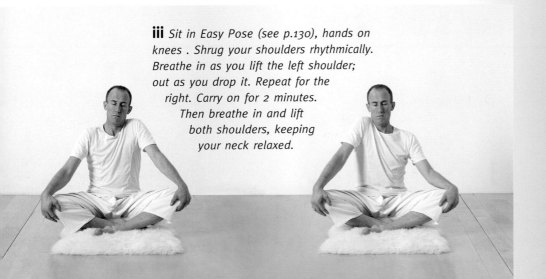

ii *Sit in Rock Pose (see p.132), eyes closed. Extend both arms, parallel to the ground.*

Turn your head to the left while breathing in deeply. Turn your head to the right while breathing out deeply. Mentally breathe in "Sat" and breathe out "Nam". Continue for 3 minutes.

iii *Sit in Easy Pose (see p.130), hands on knees . Shrug your shoulders rhythmically. Breathe in as you lift the left shoulder; out as you drop it. Repeat for the right. Carry on for 2 minutes. Then breathe in and lift both shoulders, keeping your neck relaxed.*

iv *Sit in Rock Pose (see p.132). Extend your arms, palms down. Let your head drop back and look up. Begin Breath of Fire (see p.120). Carry on for 3 minutes. Then breathe in, straighten your neck, and pull in your chin. Relax.*

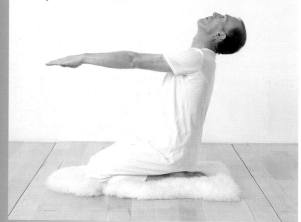

v *Sit in Easy Pose (see p.130), hands in Venus Lock (see p.127) behind the small of the back. Tilt your head forwards. Begin Breath of Fire (see p.120) and carry on for 3 minutes.*

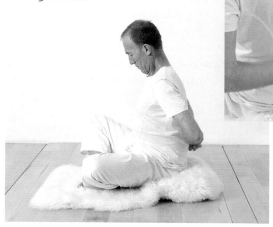

vi *Sit in Easy Pose, chest slightly lifted. Rest your hands on the knees in Gyan Mudra (see p.126). Breathe in completely, turning your head to the right. Breathe out totally, turning it to the left. Mentally vibrate "Sat Nam". Continue for 26 breaths. Breathe in to the center at the end and hold for a few moments as you focus at the Third Eye.*

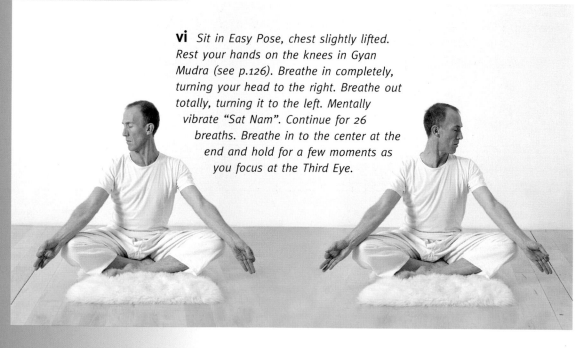

vii *With eyes open, sit with legs extended, together. Press your feet forwards. Place your hands behind. Lean back 30 degrees, lift your head up and back. Start a regular, long, deep breath and carry on for 5 minutes. Then breathe in and straighten the neck. Relax.*

Yogi Bhajan comments:
This set is a complete workout for the thyroid and parathyroid glands. ... Do this kriya every day for 40 days, at the same time of day. Then chant "Sat Nam Sat Nam Sat Nam Sat Nam Sat Nam Sat Nam Sat Nam Wahe Guru". ... Then contemplate your words of the previous day; were they true and from the heart? Be humble, forthright, sincere, and truthful. You will understand their real meaning. You will increase your sensitivity to speak what is true. Your word will gain force with yourself and with others.

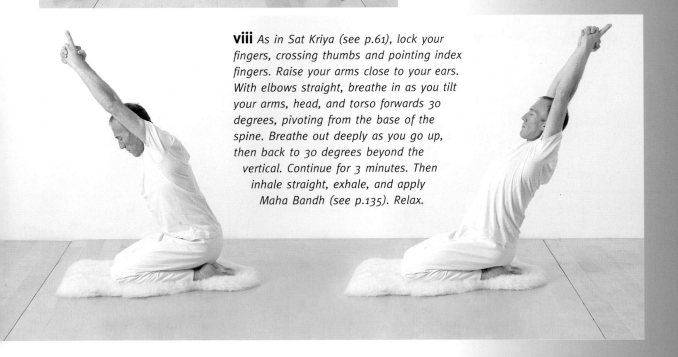

viii *As in Sat Kriya (see p.61), lock your fingers, crossing thumbs and pointing index fingers. Raise your arms close to your ears. With elbows straight, breathe in as you tilt your arms, head, and torso forwards 30 degrees, pivoting from the base of the spine. Breathe out deeply as you go up, then back to 30 degrees beyond the vertical. Continue for 3 minutes. Then inhale straight, exhale, and apply Maha Bandh (see p.135). Relax.*

Sixth Chakra
AJNA

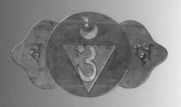

i *Adopt Virasan by sitting on your left heel, right foot on the floor, palms together. Stretch your left arm out at 60 degrees, and move your left hand up and down at the wrist as rapidly as you can. Coordinate the movement with Breath of Fire (see p.120) for 3 minutes. Swap arms and continue for 3 minutes. Swap arms again and carry on for 3 minutes. Finally, stretch out both arms and restart with both arms for 2 minutes. Shut your eyes and imagine yourself flying. Move through the 5 elements and identify with each one — Ether, Air, Fire, Water, Earth, and Ether again. Sense the differences. Spend about 15 seconds on each.*

6a Kriya for the Sixth Chakra

Originally taught by Yogi Bhajan as
SYNCHRONIZE THE BRAIN AND BALANCE THE TATTVAS in 1985

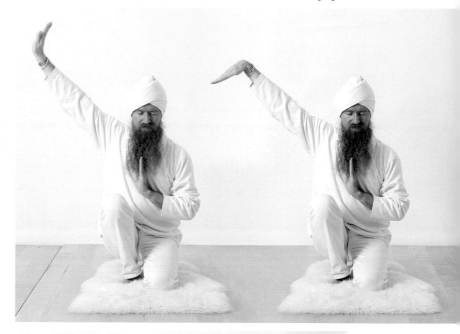

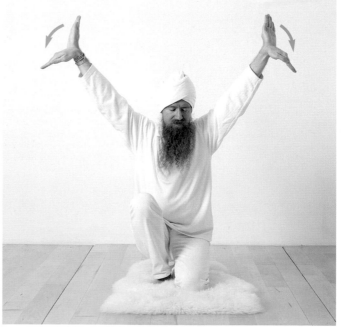

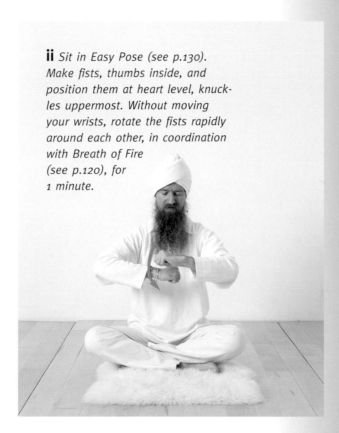

ii *Sit in Easy Pose (see p.130). Make fists, thumbs inside, and position them at heart level, knuckles uppermost. Without moving your wrists, rotate the fists rapidly around each other, in coordination with Breath of Fire (see p.120), for 1 minute.*

Yogi Bhajan comments:

All living matter comprises five elements: Earth, Air, Fire, Water, and Ether. These are the five tattvas. Practice of this kriya will bring the tattvas into balance, synchronizing the hemispheres of the brain. The first exercise helps differentiate the left from right hemisphere. Normally Breath of Fire creates a neutral state; here, however, hand movement creates a differentiation and synchronizes the hemispheres as well.

6b Kriya for the Sixth Chakra

Originally taught by Yogi Bhajan as AJNA STIMULATION KRIYA

i *Stand straight and tuck your thumbs inside tight fists, arms hanging. Let your head fall back and gaze at a fixed point. Breathe in and begin Breath of Fire (see p.120). Carry on for 2 to 3 minutes. Then breathe in deeply as you slowly tuck your chin in. Hold your breath briefly with your head straight. Then breathe out and relax.*
• Sets the magnetic field and opens circulation to the head.

ii *Take up Triangle Pose (see p.133). Your head is in line with your body and your arms are about 60 cm (2 ft) apart. Take long, deep breaths for 2 to 3 minutes. Then breathe in. Breathe out and apply Mul Bandh, or Root Lock (see p.134). Hold the breath out briefly. Breathe in and relax.*
• Aids digestion and strengthens the nervous system.

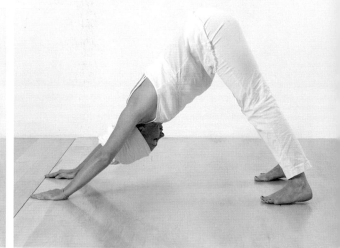

iii *Take up Bow Pose (see p.128). Breathe in and arch your spine, pulling on your ankles, pelvis, abdomen, lower chest staying in contact with the ground. Tilt your head back and take long, deep breaths for 1 to 3 minutes. Then breathe in, gently stretching the spine. Breathe out and relax.*
• Aids digestion and opens the central nerve channel.

iv *Take up Stretch Pose (see p.132). Extend your arms and lift your head and shoulders 15 cm (6 in). Gaze towards your toes. Begin Breath of Fire (see p.120) and continue for 1 to 3 minutes. Breathe in and hold briefly. Breathe out and relax.*
• Activates and balances the energy of the Third Chakra, sets the Navel Point, and tones the abdominal muscles.

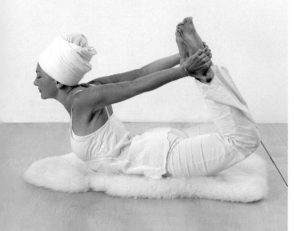

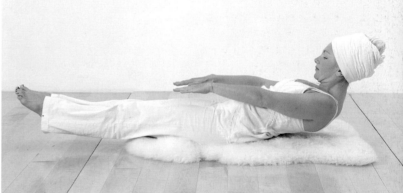

v *Sit on your heels. Keeping your head straight and shoulders relaxed, breathe in and flex your upper body as far forward as you can. Arms rest on your knees. As you breathe out flex back the other way. Begin slowly and continue rhythmically with the breath for 1 to 3 minutes. To finish, breathe out and relax.*
• Prepares the spine for step **vi**.

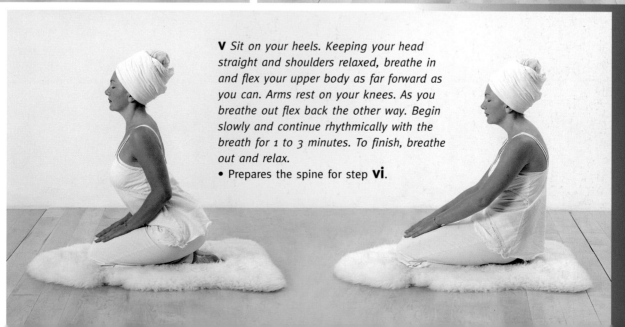

vi *Sit on your heels and part your knees wide. Lower your forehead to the ground, palms resting on soles. Focus at the Third Eye and relax, while breathing normally. Continue for 5 to 20 minutes. Take a few deep breaths and gradually release. NB Always follow this exercise with Bundle Roll (see below and p.129).*
• Subtly uses the sexual energy of the Second Chakra to stimulate the Sixth.

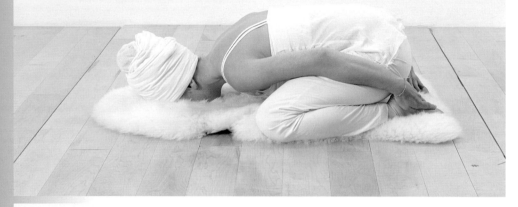

vii *Do Bundle Roll (see also p.129) for 3 to 5 minutes. Then relax.*
• Balances the magnetic field and massages the muscles.

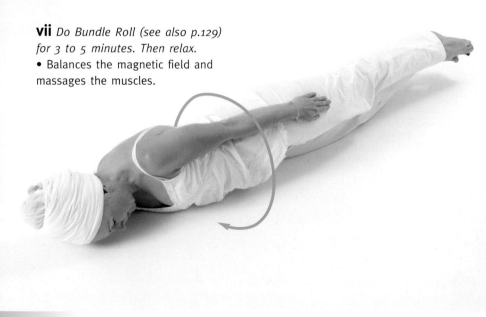

viii *Sit with spine straight, hands in Gyan Mudra (see p.126). Lock your chin, so your head is straight on your spine, and breathe in deeply. As you breathe out, chant "Sat" (extending the sound and dividing it into 7 undulations, each of 5 beats, for a total of 35 beats). Complete the breathing out by chanting "Nam" for one beat. Then breathe in and repeat. Chant from your heart, visualizing the sound spiralling up your spine and out the top of your head. Continue for at least 3 minutes before breathing in. Hold briefly, then breath out and relax.*
• A call to balance your energy and lead your consciousness to its primal Source.

ix *Relax deeply.*

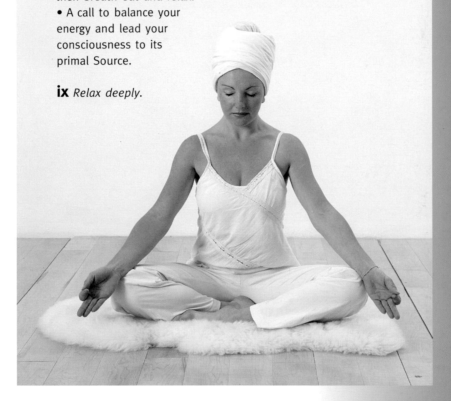

Sa a a a a a at nam

Seventh Chakra
SAHASRARA

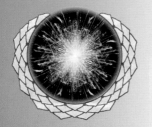

7a Kriya for the Seventh Chakra

Originally taught by Yogi Bhajan as TO EXALT THE SELF in 1985

i *Get on to your hands and knees and kick your legs straight up behind, like a donkey.*
• Energizes the brain, with the added benefit, for women, of affecting the clitoris, which in turn affects the pituitary and pineal glands, the brain, the spinal column, and, consequently, sexual activity.

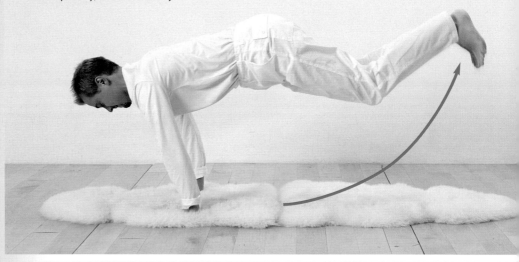

ii *Lie on your back, eyes closed, and stretch your arms above your head. Breathe in as you sit up and touch your toes. Breathe out as you return to the original position. Do the cycle 27 times.*

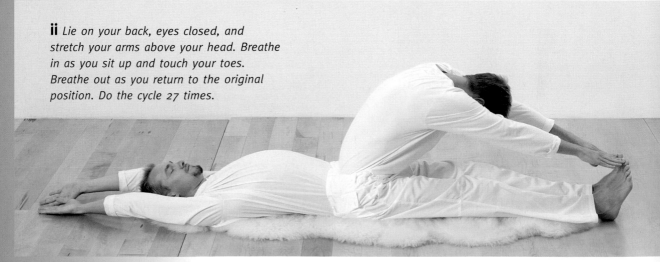

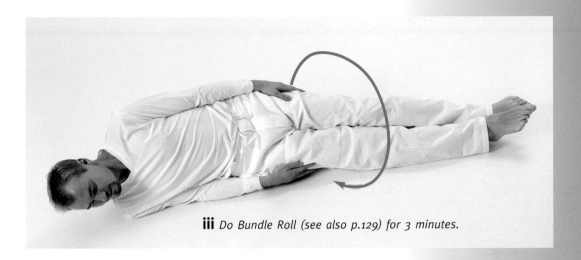

iii *Do Bundle Roll (see also p.129) for 3 minutes.*

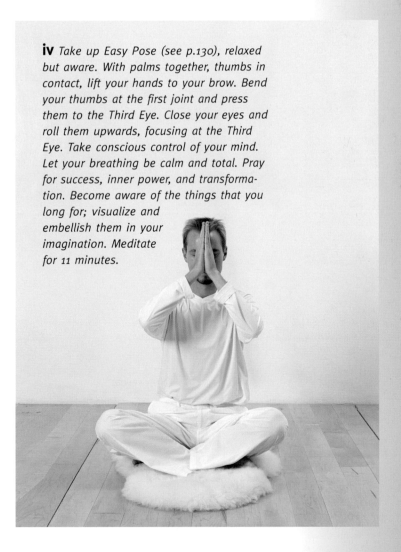

iv *Take up Easy Pose (see p.130), relaxed but aware. With palms together, thumbs in contact, lift your hands to your brow. Bend your thumbs at the first joint and press them to the Third Eye. Close your eyes and roll them upwards, focusing at the Third Eye. Take conscious control of your mind. Let your breathing be calm and total. Pray for success, inner power, and transformation. Become aware of the things that you long for; visualize and embellish them in your imagination. Meditate for 11 minutes.*

V *Sit in Easy Pose (see p.130), elbows held in to your body. Hold your forearms at a 60-degree angle. The hands are horizontal with palms up. Meditate for 6 minutes.*
•Your inner state is of prayerful awareness. Be prepared to receive the guidance, offerings, and protection of the Cosmos. Feel the energy from your palms.

vi *Hold your crossed-over hands to your chest. Meditate using concentration and prayer. Assume the posture of the Exalted Self within you. God and all the deities acknowledge you. Your prayer is powerful and you can count on miracles. You are in connection with all that exists. Be an expanded being and full of peace. Continue for 11 to 31 minutes.*

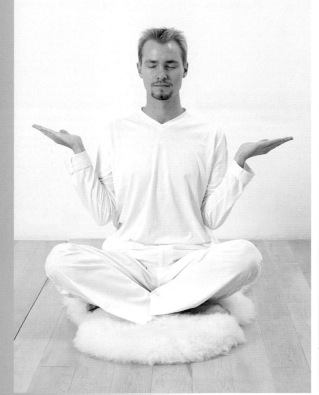

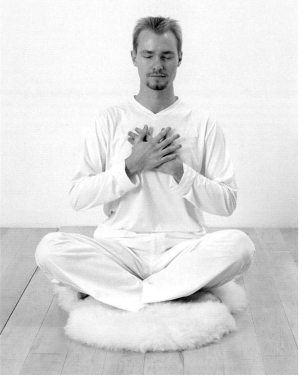

Yogi Bhajan comments:

Do this kriya to command, integrate, and exalt yourself. Find the observing center of intuition inside. It gives you the power to choose and act from your Exalted Self, regardless of the vicissitudes of the five elements. This kriya stimulates sexual energy, the sympathetic and parasympathetic systems, and the pituitary and the pineal glands, while strengthening the digestive system and the magnetic field.

7b Kriya for the Seventh Chakra

Originally taught by Yogi Bhajan as FOUNDATION FOR INFINITY in 1985

i *Eyes closed, sit in Easy Pose (see p.130) hands interlaced at your hairline. Keeping your upper arms parallel to the ground, breathe in and rotate to the left, then breathe out and rotate to the right. Continue at moderate pace for 3 minutes.*

ii *In Easy Pose, interlace the hands behind the base of the spine. Begin Breath of Fire (see p.120) and bend forwards into Yoga Mudra (see p.133). Continue to alternate positions at a steady pace for 2 minutes.*

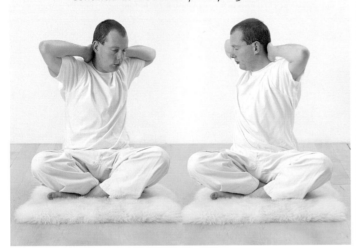

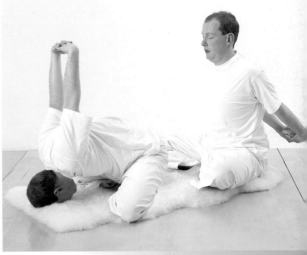

iii *Take up Back Platform pose (see p.128), head dropped back. Lower your buttocks to the ground and align your head with your spine. Create a regular tempo, alternating with Breath of Fire (see p.120) for 1½ minutes.*
• Increases the strength and flexibility of the pelvic area and releases the pelvis if it is locked.

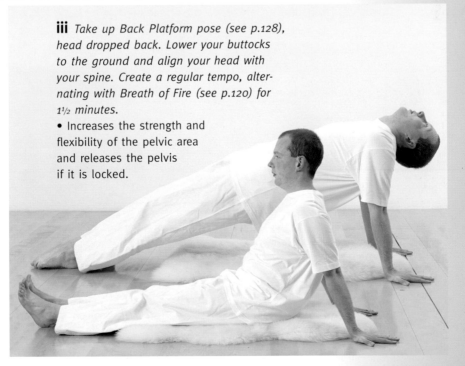

iv *Squat in Crow Pose (see p.130) and extend your arms, palms down, parallel to the ground. Breathe in and stand, breathe out, and squat down. Repeat the cycle 52 times (26 squats).*

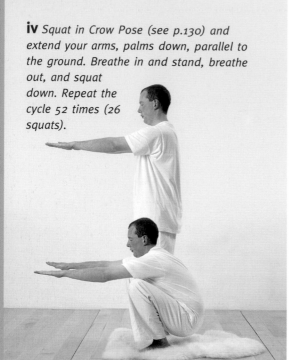

v *Stand with legs shoulder-width apart. Stretch your arms up. Breathe in and stretch back as far as possible, then breathe out and bend to touch the ground. Repeat the cycle 26 times.*

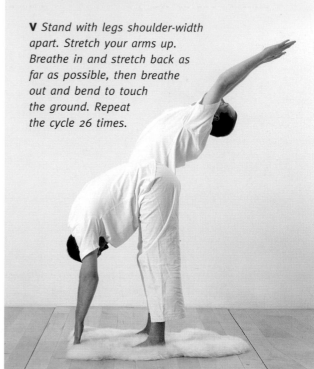

vi *Stand straight and stretch your arms above your head. Breathe in and bend to the left, then breathe out and bend to the right. Bend to each side 26 times, then relax your arms.*

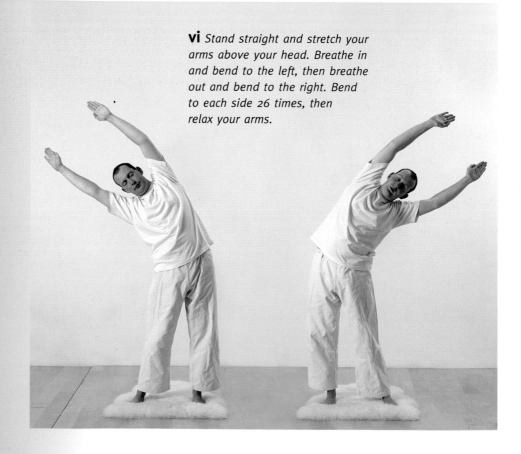

vii *Put your hands on your hips and kick alternate legs forwards, keeping them straight. With each kick chant "Har", putting your tongue tip on your palate on the "r" sound. Kick once per second, for 3 minutes.*

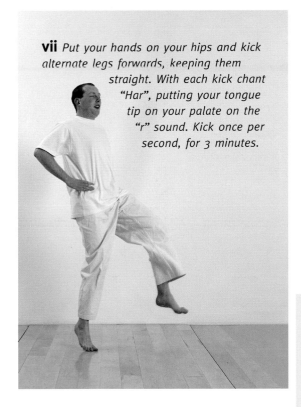

viii *Sit in Easy Pose (see p.130). Put your hands in your lap, right palm in left, thumb pads touching. Turn the eyes up and focus on the Seventh Chakra. Mentally say "Har Har", pulling your Navel Point in. Pressing your tongue tip to the roof of your mouth, pull the navel again and mentally say "Mukanday". Go within. Discover the shining light of Sahasrara (Seventh Chakra). Find you are never-ending. Go beyond time and space, into total harmony and happiness. Continue for 11 to 31 minutes.*

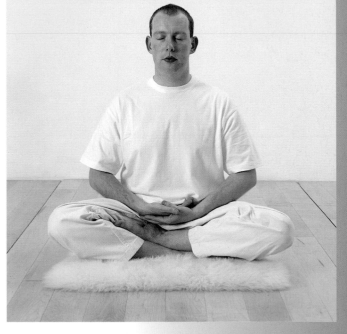

Yogi Bhajan comments:
To reach the subtle realm of Ether, where you are boundless, first set a firm foundation on Earth. Practicing this kriya is a means of setting that foundation. Then the meditation launches you into the realms of Infinity. The pelvis acts as a foundation for the torso and lower body. The female pelvis can be easily misaligned. Chronic mis-alignment, tension, and inflexibility will eventually manifest through impotency, sciatica, and menstrual irregularities.

Meditation for the Soul Body

1a Originally taught by Yogi Bhajan as KUNDALINI MEDITATION on 22nd November 1977

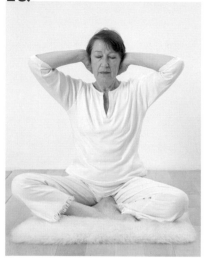

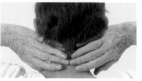

Sit in Easy Pose (see p.130), eyes almost closed. Place your hands over your ears, middle fingers touching. Your little fingers and palm edges touch the base of your skull. Spread your arms wide. Inhale and exhale deeply several times, in preparation. Then breathe in and chant "Ek Ong Kara" (see p.122) powerfully, using all your breath. Breathe in and repeat the chant once more. Repeat this cycle again. After finishing the third cycle press your tongue flat against the upper palate, with all your strength, for 60 seconds. Go back to normal breathing for the next minute.

NB Do not do this mantra more than 3 consecutive times, or keep your tongue pressed for more than a minute.

1b Originally taught by Yogi Bhajan as THREE MEDITATIONS FOR THE HEART CENTER on 4th April 1972

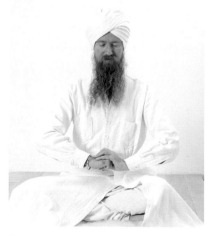

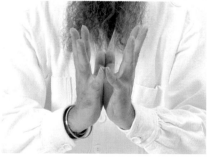

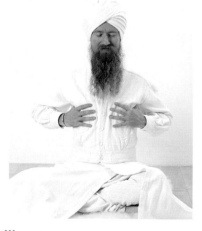

i *In Easy Pose (see p.130), make your right hand a fist, thumb out-stretched. Hold your fist with your left hand and press your right thumb into your navel. Breathe long and deep. Concentrate on your breath. Notice the breath pulse between navel and nose root. Continue for 11 minutes.*

ii *Put your hands in Lotus Mudra (see p.126), 10 or 12 cm (4 or 5 in) in front of your Heart Center. Commence long, deep, slow breathing. Pull your chin in, without inclining your head, and gaze at your thumbtips. Feel your breath contact your thumbs. Continue for 11 minutes.*

iii *Apply pressure to the nerve in your armpit by inserting your thumbs and bringing your elbows to your sides, palms on chest. Breathe in with a whistle. Mentally hear "So". Breathe out through the nose and hear "Hung" — "I am that Infinite". Continue for 11 minutes.*

Meditation for the Negative Mind

2a Originally taught by Yogi Bhajan as HARI SHABAD MEDITATION on 14th July 1978

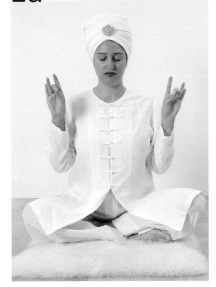

Sit in Easy Pose (see p.130), pulling your chin in and pushing your chest out. Hold your elbows into your body and lift your fore-arms 30 degrees forwards from upright. Your fingers form Shuni Mudra (see p.127). Your eyes remain one-tenth open.

Breathe in deeply and chant "Sat Nam, Haree Nam, Haree Nam, Haree. Haree Nam Sat Nam Sat Nam Haree" three times as you breathe out. Carry on for 31 minutes. Then chant "Sa-a-a-a-at Nam" (making "Sat" 8 times longer than "Nam") for 3 minutes. Finally

chant "Guru Guru, Wahe Guru, Guru Ram Das Guru" for 3 minutes in a monotone, emphasizing the first syllable of each word.

Yogi Bhajan comments:
"Haree" is the creative energy of God. "Sat Nam" explodes it; it is the higher potency and multiplies the power of "Haree" millions of times.

2b Originally taught by Yogi Bhajan as HEALING MEDITATION FOR ACUTE DEPRESSION on 9th February 1976

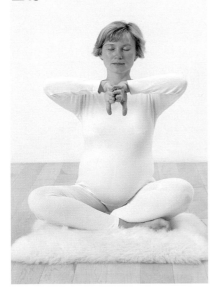

Sit in Easy Pose (see p.130) and place your hands 15 cm (6 in) from the chest in Reverse Prayer Mudra (see. p.127), creating tension on the backs of the hands. Focus your eyes on the tip of your nose. Breathe in and out deeply several times to prepare. Breathe in deeply and chant "Wahay Guru" 16 times as you breathe out. One complete cycle will take 20–25 seconds. Continue for 11 minutes, building gradually to 31 minutes.

Meditation for the Positive Mind

3a

Originally taught by Yogi Bhajan as MEDITATION TO RELAX AND REJOICE on 18th January 1979

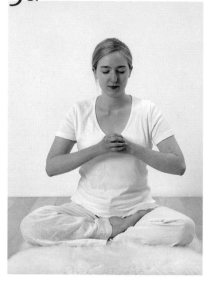

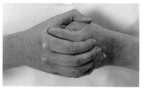

Yogi Bhajan comments:
This helps you appreciate the contrast between working from your ego and from your inner self, the will of God, the soul.

Adopt Easy Pose (see p.130). Relax. Bring your hands together just above your solar plexus. Make a fist around your left thumb, your right thumb on top of the base of your left thumb and your right hand around your left fist. Focus on the tip of your nose. Breathe in deeply, and then out completely as you chant in a monotone, "Haree Har Haree Har Haree Har Haree Har Haree Har Haree Har Haree Har Haree Har". Continue for 11 minutes, building gradually to 62.*

3b

Originally taught by Yogi Bhajan as ANTI-DEPRESSION & BRAIN SYNCHRONY MEDITATION

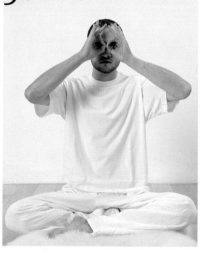

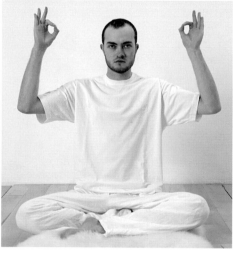

Yogi Bhajan comments:
This meditation will let you evaluate how positive or negative you are and will make you positive and happy. It focuses on the range of the breath. In the subconscious, breath and life are synonymous. By meditating this way, you can alleviate depression. If you do it correctly, there will be tremendous pressure at the lymph glands.

Assume Easy Pose (see p.130), with your hands in Gyan Mudra (see p.126). Raise your arms and look through the rings. Stare into Infinity. Keeping your upper arms horizontal, breathe in deeply and bring your lower arms to the vertical, mentally chanting "Sa". Breathe out, moving back to the first position, mentally chanting "Ta". Breathe in and bring your lower arms to the vertical, mentally chanting "Na". Exhale, moving back to the first position, mentally chanting "Ma". This cycle takes about 4 seconds. Meditate on the prana in the breath. Feel you are stretching the breath from a single point to the* width of your arms. After 3 minutes, increase speed to 3½ seconds for each cycle of "Sa-Ta-Na-Ma", and continue for 3 more minutes. Then breathe in and relax the arms. Focus on the point just in front of the center of the top of the skull, totally relaxing it. Continue for 15 minutes.*

Meditation for the Neutral Mind

4a Originally taught by Yogi Bhajan as THREE-MINUTE KRIYA TO DEVELOP A MEDITATIVE MIND on 1st December 1977

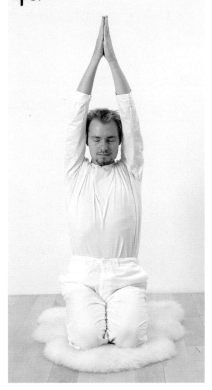

Sit in Rock Pose (see p.132). Stretch your arms, pressing palms together with fingers and thumbs together, pointing straight. Lock your elbows, upper arms against your ears. Your eyes are one-tenth open. Focus on the breath. Breathe in and out deeply several times to prepare. Breathe in slowly and deeply, hold the breath as long as you can, and then breathe out completely. This breathing in and holding the breath should last 60 seconds. Repeat twice more.

Yogi Bhajan comments:
This meditation is one of several that can develop a meditative mind, with practice. This gives you the intuitive ability to realize the consequences of a sequence of actions and therefore gives guidelines for dealing with cause and effect and minimizing karma.

4b Originally taught by Yogi Bhajan as CHOKE MEDITATION on 31st July 1975

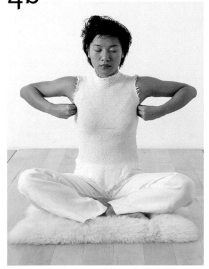

Sit in Easy Pose (see p.130). Tuck your chin in slightly and push your sternum forwards. Put your fingers into your armpits in Praying Mantis Mudra (see p.127). Close your eyes and focus on your Third Eye. Chant "Ra Ma Da Sa Sa Say So Hung". Continue for 11 minutes, gradually building to 31 minutes.

Yogi Bhajan comments:
This will work on your inner faculty and your ego, which is revealed by five things: two legs, two hands, and one tongue. No investigator can penetrate you if you can control these five organs. ... Your metabolism will go through a tremendous change in this meditation, which is like a bitter melon. The discomfort it creates is all in the head. It brings the combination of the five centers of the left and right brain into the neutral self.

Meditation for the Physical Body

5a
Originally taught by Yogi Bhajan as MEDITATION INTO BEING on 7th April 1972

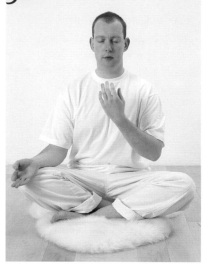

Sit in Easy Pose (see p.130), resting your right wrist on your knee. Place your left hand, palm inward, 15 cm (6 in) in front of your chest, at heart level. Move the hand to 10 cm (4 in) from the chest and say "I am", then move it 30 cm (12 in) out from your chest and say "I am". Breathe in and bring your hand to the original 15-cm (6-in) position. Carry on this cycle for 11 minutes. Slowly increase the time to 31 minutes.

Yogi Bhajan comments:
The mantra "I am, I am" relates the finite identity of the first "I am" with the infinite identity of the second one. If you say "I am" in your mind, immediately the mind asks "What?" If you say only one "I am", you will try to answer "I am what?" This produces a finite identity and does not expand the mind beyond the limited self. But if you immediately say a second "I am", the thought becomes "I am what I am", and to be what you are is the essence of truth. Each time the hand moves, extend yourself beyond the body's physical limits.

5b
Originally taught by Yogi Bhajan as a KUNDALINI MEDITATION on 15th September 1977

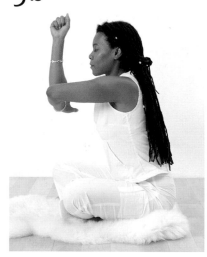

Sit in Easy Pose (see p.130). Lean forwards 30 degrees. Make your right hand a tight fist and raise your right arm so that the lower arm is vertical and the upper arm horizontal. Your lower left arm and hand are horizontal, with the back of your left hand touching the bottom of your right elbow. Close your eyes. Breathe in deeply and breathe out completely several times, to prepare. Then breathe in deeply and breathe out completely by chanting 3 times, "Satanam Satanam Satanam Satanam Satanam Satanam Wahe Guru". Continue for 7 minutes.
Then chant 4 times per breath "Healthy am I, Happy am I, Holy am I". Continue for 4 minutes. To finish, breathe in deeply and hold. Breathe out completely and relax.

Yogi Bhajan comments:
This meditation produces heat, so it is good to practice it in a cool place. If it is practiced for 11 minutes a day, it contributes to your well-being. Any restlessness will be released. The mudras allow the astral body to help the balancing process. In this way, you don't leave the body.

Meditation for the Arc Line

6a

Originally taught by Yogi Bhajan as DHRIB DHRISTI LOCHINA KARMA KRIYA on 10th October 1973

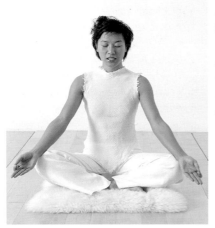

Sit in Easy Pose (see p.130). Bite the tips of the front teeth together. Touch the tongue to the upper palate and focus the eyes on the tip of the nose. Mentally project the mantra "Sa Ta Na Ma" out from the Third Eye for 31 minutes. (The minimum time is 15 minutes.)

Yogi Bhajan comments:
Dhrib Dhristi Lochina Karma Kriya is the action of acquiring the insight of the future. Its effect on the subconscious mind will be heightened if practiced on the full Moon. Mastery of this practice brings the power to heal with your eyes and inspire with your words. You will be able to project your personality and to know the effect of any cause you begin.

6b

Originally taught by Yogi Bhajan as MEDITATION FOR THE ARC LINE AND TO CLEAR THE KARMAS on 1st August 1996

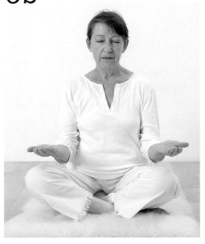
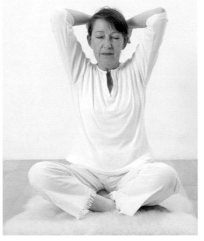

Yogi Bhajan comments:
This meditation is for the Arc Line and to clear karma stored there. Wahe Guru is just a hand of prayer. Remember, the power of Infinity is not outside, it is inside. When "I" and Infinity create impact, you'll become totally Divine. Otherwise there's a duality that keeps you away from reality.

i *Sit in Easy Pose (see p.130), eyes closed. Drop your elbows, holding forearms out, parallel to the ground, palms flat. Then cup your palms slightly, and hold them above your knees.*
ii *Move your arms behind your head, stretching your arms as far over your shoulders as possible.*

Visualize scooping up water and casting it through your Arc Line, over your shoulders, by flicking your wrists. The action is seamless and rhythmic. Carry on at 4 scoops to 10 seconds chanting "Wahay Guru, Wahay Guru, Wahay Guru, Wahay Jeeo" for 3–31 minutes. Do one complete round per repetition

of the mantra; scooping up, throwing, and coming back to the starting point.
iii *To complete, breathe in, and stretch your hands back as far as possible. Hold 10–15 seconds. Breathe out. Repeat 3 times total. Relax.*

Meditation for the Aura

7a   Originally taught by Yogi Bhajan as MEDITATION FOR GURPRASAD

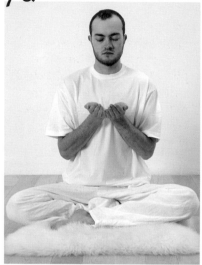

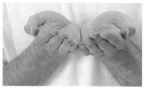

Sit in Easy Pose (see p.130). Make your hands into cups. Press your upper arms against your ribs and bring your hands to heart level. Your eyes begin one-tenth open and close during the meditation. Go beyond words and ask for a blessing from God. Your breath will adjust itself. Meditate on the Divine flow and feel the spirit move. Continue until this happens. Practice for as long as you like.

Yogi Bhajan comments:
This is a very restful posture. The subtle pressure against the meridian points on the rib cage give immediate relaxation. As you practice, feel yourself showered by all the blessings of heaven: health, wealth, happiness, your ultimate calibre, and capacity. Fill your heart and soul with all the bounties of Nature.

7b   Originally taught by Yogi Bhajan as MEDITATION FOR THE DIVINE SHIELD on 24th September 1971

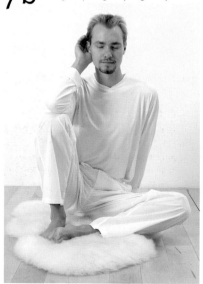

Sit with right knee upright and left on the ground. With the sole of your left foot push into your right foot, the ball just in front of your right anklebone. Lean back on your left fist. Place your right elbow on your right knee, the palm of your right hand cupping your ear. Breathe in deeply and begin chanting a long, smooth "Ma", listening through your cupped palm. Continue for 3–31 minutes, then change sides and continue for the same duration.

Yogi Bhajan comments:
Your fundamental nature is to unfold. Fear curtails this and you become unhappy. If you are fear-less, your potential will unfold. This ... meditation calls on the Cosmos, or God, through the sound of com-passion and stimulates the inner sounds. The Universe becomes the mother and you the child. Call and She shall come to your aid.

8 *Meditation for the Pranic Body*

8a Originally taught by Yogi Bhajan as MEDITATION FOR A STABLE BODY on 27th September 1979

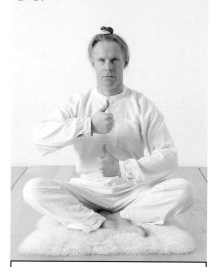

This meditation could not be verified by KRI and therefore is not certified as accurate. (See website address p.143.)

Sit in Easy Pose (see p.130). Make fists 12 cm (5 in) in front of the throat, thumbs upwards. Align the thumbs, with the tip of the left one 5 cm (2 in) below the base of the right hand. Forearms are parallel to the Earth. The eyes are one-tenth open and focus at Third Eye. Apply Jalandhara Bandh, or Neck Lock (see p.135). Inhale sharply and deeply, exhale powerfully and completely. Hold the breath out and rhythmically apply Mul Bandh, or Root Lock (see p.134) 26 times. As you hold the breath visualize energy moving from the base of the spine to the center of the head. Continue for 11 minutes.

Yogi Bhajan comments:
Do not exceed 11 minutes. Overcome the concerns of the physical body. The concentration must be held and the visualization perfected. Complete stability of the Pranic Body will be achieved. Subconscious fears affect our judgement and this meditation removes the reactions of fear and makes you steady.

8b Originally taught by Yogi Bhajan as MEDITATION TO TAKE THE FINITE TO THE INFINITE on 2nd October 1972

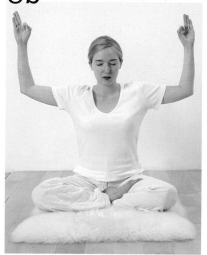

Sit in Easy Pose (see p.130), hands in Gyan Mudra (see p.126). Stretch your arms out at shoulder level, upper arms horizontal, and lower arms to the vertical. Focus at the Third Eye. Chant "Wa Hay Gu Ru" slowly and rhythmically (4 distinct sounds). Continue for 11 minutes, gradually increasing to 31 minutes.

Yogi Bhajan comments:
... If you want to live for something, live for Infinity. The Infinite is an unknown totality, while the known is individuality. Achieving neutrality will lead you through the times.

Meditation for the Subtle Body

9a
Originally taught by Yogi Bhajan in the MAN-TO-MAN LECTURES

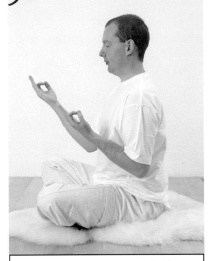

This meditation could not be verified by KRI and therefore is not certified as accurate. (See website address p.143.)

Sit in Easy Pose (see p.130), hands in Gyan Mudra (see p.126), elbows at your sides, forearms 45 degrees to the vertical. Your right arm is a hand's length further forwards than the left. Visualize walking barefoot on grass at dawn. Be open to your senses. Notice the sky lightening. You are connecting with a morning star. Repeat silently "I am Light". Imagine a shaft of light from the star connecting to your Heart Chakra. Feel the rays turn into a path of light upon which you can walk. Feel your feet on the path of light. Feel yourself walking up to the stars. Your body becomes more relaxed and lighter; your awareness more subtle. Carry on walking and mentally repeat "I am Light". Merge with the Light. Breathe in deeply, hold it, and become one with the Light. Experience the breath and the Light, the inner and the outer, as one. Slowly breathe out. Repeat several times, holding your breath as long as possible. Imagine yourself lying on the grass gazing up at the early morning sky and begin to stretch into wakefulness.

Yogi Bhajan comments:
This posture gives you the power to transfer yourself into the Subtle Body, which gives you the power to walk on Light.

9b
Originally taught by Yogi Bhajan as YONI KRIYA MEDITATION on 27th March 1979

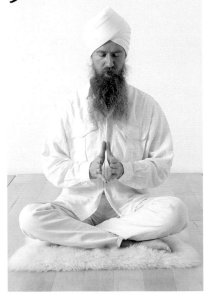

Sit in Easy Pose (see p.130). Place the hands in Yoni Mudra variation (see p.127) at the solar plexus. The tips of the little fingers touch and point forwards, thumbs touching and arching back towards the chest. The other fingers are parallel to the Earth and to each other and as far apart as possible. The eyes are focused on the tip of the nose. Pucker the lips as if blowing a kiss. Inhale fully through the nose. Exhale completely through the mouth. Inhale fully through the mouth. Exhale completely through the nose. Continue for 3 minutes, gradually building to 11 minutes. To end: inhale deeply through the nose, turn the eyes up to the crown, and hold in stillness for 30 seconds. Exhale and relax.

Yogi Bhajan comments:
Yoni refers to both the female sexual organ and to the cavity at the base of the spine that holds the Kundalini. In this mudra the open space between the hands is the yoni: the cave of creativity. The thumbs represent the male organ and the three fingers past, present, and future.

The fruit of this subtle union is born outside time and space and has the potential to neutralize the karmic patterns of our actions within time and space. It may be beneficial to practice it at night before sleeping.

Meditation for the Radiant Body

10a

Originally taught by Yogi Bhajan as MEDITATION TO MAKE YOU FEEL COSY AND CONTENTED on 29th September 1975

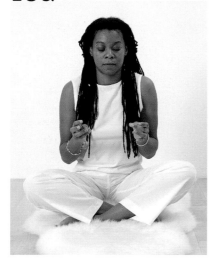

Sit in Easy Pose (see p.130). For women, your left hand is in Shuni Mudra (see p.127), your right hand in Buddhi Mudra (see p.126). For men, vice versa. Make sure that your fingernails do not touch. Place your hands 15–17 cm (7–8 in) apart, fingers forwards and 7–10 cm (3–4 in) in front of your nipples. Your shoulders are relaxed and your eyes one-tenth open. Let your breath regulate itself. Meditate for 11 minutes. To finish, breathe in, make tight fists and hold, squeezing even tighter, for 10 seconds, before breathing out and relaxing.

Yogi Bhajan comments:
This meditation makes you feel cosy and contented. It balances the brain by reinforcing your ability to be in continual touch with your Higher Self.

10b

Originally taught by Yogi Bhajan as MEDITATION TO BRIGHTEN YOUR RADIANCE on 23rd July 1996

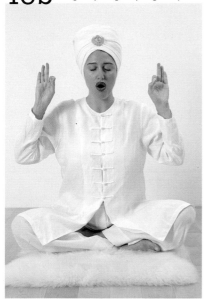

Sit in Easy Pose (see p.130), your hands 30 cm (12 in) either side of your ears with the index fingers curled under the thumb in a variation of Gyan Mudra (see p.126). Keep your elbows down. Focus on the tip of your nose. Make your mouth an "o" and breathe long and deep. Hold the position for 11–31 minutes. To finish, breathe in deeply, hold, come into a state of Shuniaa (zero), and synchronize your entire being. Hold for 20 seconds.

Yogi Bhajan comments:
You are known by your spirit. You project out by your radiance. You are loved and honoured by your excellence or stupidity. Who are you? You are a "hu-man being". "Hu" means spirit, the light, the hue. "Man" means now, mental, being now. Now you are the spirit of your mind. You are a bright light of yourself. That's your identity.

Meditation for the Embodiment

11a Originally taught by Yogi Bhajan as COMMANDING THE COMMAND CENTER OF THE GLANDULAR SYSTEM on 19th May 1993

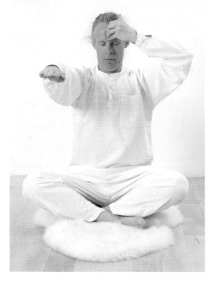

i *Sit in Easy Pose (see p.130). Stretch your right arm forwards, palm down. Raise your left arm at shoulder level, elbow bent. Rest the fingertips on your forehead in a line between hairline and base of your nose, thumb pointing straight up. Close your eyes and pump your navel rapidly with Breath of Fire (see p.120) for 3 minutes.*
To finish, breathe in deeply, breathe out, hold your breath out for 10 seconds, squeeze all your muscles and breathe in. Repeat twice more and relax.

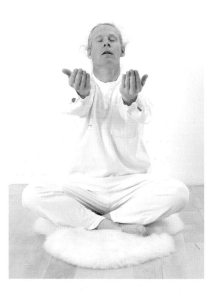

ii *Stretch your arms out, without locking your elbows. With palms up cup your hands. Open your mouth, tilt your head back, relaxing your lips, teeth, and tongue. Pump your navel vigorously for 3 minutes. To finish, breathe in and, holding the breath for 20 seconds, lock your back teeth together and tighten your jaw. Breathe out and repeat twice more. Relax.*

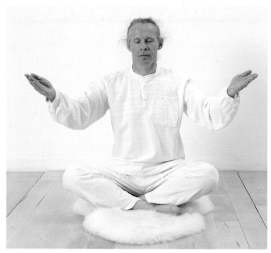

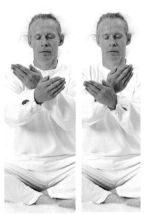

Yogi Bhajan comments:
*Exercise **i** powerfully cleans out the subconscious mind. Your whole body must shake with the power of the navel movement.*
*Exercise **ii** puts a pressure on the third and fourth vertebrae. Practicing this daily can give you the spirit to conquer death.*
*Exercise **iii** cleans the subconscious mind through stimulating the pituitary gland (responsible for intuition and projection).*

iii *Open your arms wide. Breathe in and, holding, criss-cross your hands rapidly. Each hand alternately passes above and below the other. Breathe out, breathe in, hold, and begin again. Carry on for 3 minutes. To finish, relax and sleep. Feel how quickly neurosis can leave you.*

11b Originally taught by Yogi Bhajan as LAYA YOGA ON ECSTASY

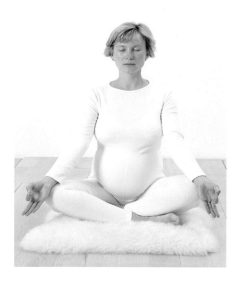

Sit in Easy Pose (see p.130), eyes closed, hands in Gyan Mudra (see p.126), elbows locked. Sit majestically, as though in the court of a king. Chant "Wahay Guru" for 11 minutes. To finish, inhale and hold your breath for 30 seconds, focusing on the crown of the head. Exhale and relax.

Yogi Bhajan comments:
Ecstasy exists within. It is the Infinite Pool to refresh the heart, giving strength to creating a better self and world. This meditation leads to that experience. So calm, so sleepy, like the merging of a raindrop into a vast, calm lake you reflect all, cleanse all. If you can cross all, you can know the extent of living in yourself, with balanced consciousness, playing with the Infinite.

Part 4

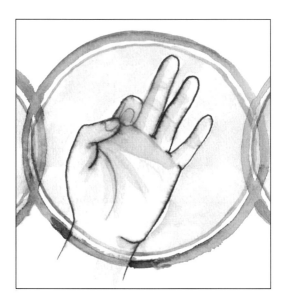

kundalini components

This section outlines important information
about the separate techniques that make
up Kundalini Yoga. They are: Breath,
Mantras, Mudras, Asanas, and Bandhs and
they are referred to constantly in Part 3
(The Kriyas and Meditations)

Breath

We need food and water to sustain life, but more essential to us than either is the breath, the real food of life. It has been said that we are what we eat, but if you change the way you breathe you change the person you are. For example, if you are frightened your breath will become shallow. This is called clavicular breathing. If you were to sustain a practice of clavicular breathing you could induce a panic attack. We respond to the breath and the breath responds to us. Conscious control of the breath is an essential part of yogic practice. The breath contains prana, or Life Force, which determines the energetic radiance, the physical health, and the psychological well-being of a person. The science of yogic breathing is called "pranayama", which means to lead or guide the Life Force. Kundalini Yoga employs a wide spectrum of breathing techniques to balance, energize, modify, and heal. The fundamental pranayama practices need to be understood and experienced to ensure safe, effective practice.

Unless otherwise instructed breathing in Kundalini Yoga is always in and out through the nose.

Long, Deep Breathing

Relax your neck and shoulders as you inhale long, slow, and deep into the abdomen. As your abdomen expands and fills, allow your chest to rise and to fully receive the complete breath. As you begin to exhale let your chest deflate before pulling your navel back towards your spine, expelling all the air. Continue this pattern. Place your palm on your abdomen and feel it expand on the inhale and contract on the exhale. Lying on your back may make this easier to begin with.
Benefits include calmness, gentle euphoria, and patience.

• The effect of rhythmic breathing in inducing changes in brainwave pattern is well known. If you slow the breath to eight breaths per minute you move into a meditative state; slow the rhythm to six breaths or less per minute and the pituitary gland is stimulated. If you slow down to four breaths per minute, or less, the pineal gland activates the Crown Chakra.

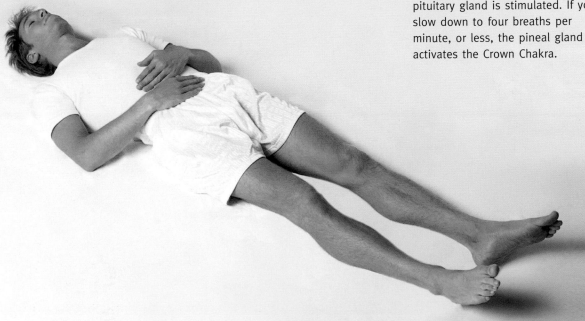

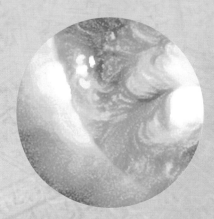

Breath of Fire

This is powerful deep breaths, done two or three times per second. You pull your navel in sharply, expelling the air. The lungs then automatically inflate as your navel is released. When learning this breath, focus on the exhale. As coordination becomes more practiced it is simple to reach the required speed of two to three breaths per second, with equal emphasis on the inhale and exhale. At first do not try to go too fast, too soon. If you find you are breathing paradoxically (back to front) try to learn to stop restricting your intake of air by pulling the navel in as you breathe in. Practice this initially lying on your back and ensure that your navel rises with the in-breath and falls with the out-breath.

• This is a powerful energizing breath, which detoxifies and balances at a core level.

Alternate Nostril Breathing

We automatically breathe through alternate nostrils, changing the primary nostril every one to two hours. Breathing through the right nostril stimulates the left side of the brain and activates your Sun energy. Breathing through the left nostril stimulates the right side of the brain and activates your Moon energy. The nostrils are the gateways of your Pranic Body, through which the prana is directed into your body. The right nostril accesses the Pingala, the positive nadi that determines your projection and energizes you. The left nostril accesses the Ida, the negative nadi that determines your receptivity and calms you.

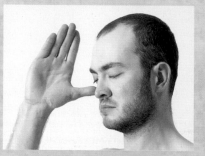

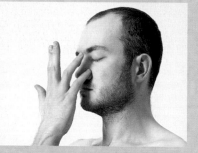

• This practice usually involves the thumb and the little finger closing alternate nostrils, while the other fingers point vertically.

Mantras

"Mantra is two words Man and Tra. Man means mind and Tra means the heat of life. Ra means Sun. So mantra is a powerful combination of words which, if recited, takes the vibratory effect of each of your molecules into the Infinity of the Cosmos."   Yogi Bhajan, 1997

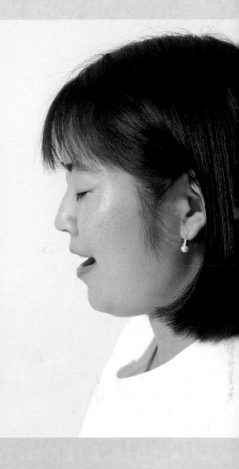

A mantra is a sound that alters, elevates, or modifies the consciousness through the repetition of its rhythm, sound, meaning, or tone. A mantra may be a single syllable, a single word, or a phrase. The most well-known mantras are from the sacred language Sanskrit, which means "perfected". Known as "the old language" throughout Asia, India, and the Orient, Sanskrit is the wellspring of mantra in the yogic, the Hindu, the Tibetan, and the Taoist traditions. The Vedas record that this creation (the Universe) was born of sound. The Sanskrit language was constructed to mirror that creation. The fifty letters of Sanskrit represent the Kulakundalini, from which derive the bij, or seed, mantras. Many of the mantras in this book are from a relatively modern form of Sanskrit called Gurmukhi.

The position of the tongue in the mouth represents a yogic science in itself. The male polarity of the tongue connects to the female polarity of the mouth at the specific point required to make the sound, completing an energy circuit and triggering a specific effect in the brain. When you chant a mantra, enunciate the movements of the mouth and tongue to derive maximum benefit.

Pronunciation guide:

a	*as in spa or baa*
ai	*as in rye or wry*
an	*as in can or tan*
ar	*as in car or jar*
ay	*as in day or play*
ee	*as in reed or redo*
o	*as in so or go*
ong	*as in gong or song*
sat	*as in but or nut*
u	*as in rue or through*
except	
gu	*short as in g'day or group*

Ong Namo Guru Dev Namo
(The Adi Mantra)
⊛

This mantra is chanted to open the link of Divinity and protection between the student and the Divine teacher. It means:

"I bow to the creative energy of the Infinite;

I bow to the Divine channel of wisdom."

Use this mantra to tune in: sit with a straight spine and join the palms together at the heart level in Prayer Pose (see p.126). Chant the Adi Mantra "Ong Namo Guru Dev Namo" once per breath and repeat at least three times. After the initial "o", which is long, as in "so" or "go", the mouth is closed and the "ng" sound resonates at the center of the head. If you are unable to chant the whole mantra on one breath, take a sip of air after "Ong Namo" and continue. The Adi Mantra invokes the golden chain of spiritual masters through the ages.

Ek Ong Kar
⊛

This mantra gives the realization that "the creator and the creation are one". It means:

"One Creator created creation."

Guru Guru Wahay Guru Guru Ram Das Guru
⊛

This ashtanga mantra invokes the presence of Guru Ram Das, who carries the mantle of Raj Yoga and who is identified as the patron saint of Kundalini Yoga. All those who respect universal service accord Guru Ram Das great reverence. It means:

"Transformation.
Ecstasy is Consciousness.
Consciousness is Serving the Infinity."

This mantra brings forth healing, energy, and protection.

Har Haray Haree
⊛

Har means "Cosmic Reality" or "the creative aspect of God". Haray means "God Projected". Hari means "God Merged".

These mantras are combined in different permutations such as:
Hari Har
Har Haray
Hari Hari Hari Har

Har Har Mukanday
⊛

Har is Cosmic Reality or the creative aspect of God. Mukanday is "that which liberates or Liberator".

Jeeo
⊛

Jeeo means "soul".

MA
※

Ma calls on the feminine mother principle; it invokes the receptive Moon energy and honours woman's capacity for birth, rebirth, and regeneration.

ONG SOHUNG
※

*Ong means "Infinite creative energy".
So Hung means "I am that".*

When you chant Ong close your mouth and vibrate the cranium and the roof of the mouth.

RA MA DA SA SA SAY SO HUNG
※

This is the Siri Gaitri Mantra. It is an ashtanga mantra containing the eight sounds of the Kundalini. It names "Sun, Moon, Earth, Infinity, All that is in Infinity, I am Thee."

SA TA NA MA
※

The syllabic form of Sat Nam. It means "Infinity, Life, Death, Rebirth".

SAT NAM
※

This is a bij, or seed, mantra. It means "Truth is my name".

SAT NAM SAT NAM SAT NAM SAT NAM SAT NAM SAT NAM WAHAY GURU
※

This is an ashtanga mantra made up of bij mantras. "Truth is my Identity, Ecstasy is Consciousness."

SAT NARAIAN WAHAY GURU HAREE NARAIAN SAT NAM
※

This mantra is chanted to create inner peace, so that one can project outer peace. Naraian embodies the element of Water. Sat Naraian is True Sustainer while Haree Naraian is Sustainer of Creation. Wahay Guru is the "Ecstasy of Consciousness" and Sat Nam is "Truth is my Name".

WAHAY GURU
※

"Ecstasy is Consciousness".

Yogi Bhajan gave the following mantras in response to requests for mantras in the English language:

GOD AND ME,
ME AND GOD,
ARE ONE

⚭

This mantra affirms a condition of elevated consciousness in triple phase.

I AM I AM

⚭

This mantra fixes your Infinite self into your psyche.

KEEP UP

⚭

The is the mantra for the Aquarian Age. You are only as good as your last thought, word, or deed.

Mudras

Mudras are the hand gestures of yoga that make subtle connections in our energetic physiology. The phrase "as above so below" encapsulates the ancients' vision that the human body is a dense physical core; a microcosmic condensation of the celestial bodies, the elements, and the planets. Mudras are used to highlight, to balance, and emphasize certain qualities of energy in the complex circuitry at the interface of the subtle, physical, and mental bodies. Physicists believe the atoms in our body derive from aeons-old stardust. Yogis hold that each of the elements and the planets manifest their influence on the physical form in specific reflex zones and they mapped the correlations between dysfunctional patterns of behaviour and imbalances in the elemental or planetary configuration of the psyche. The five fingers each represent an element, a human quality, and a planetary influence.

The following twelve mudras (see pp.126–7) are utilized in this book. They may safely be used in isolation by any experienced meditator, but obviously the effects will be enhanced when they are integrated into a Kundalini Yoga practice.

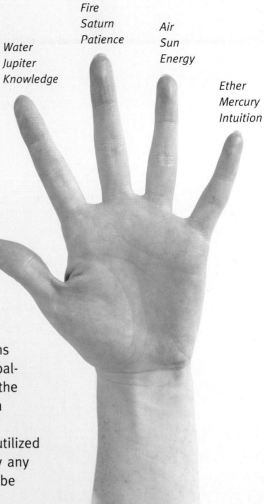

Fire
Saturn
Patience

Air
Sun
Energy

Water
Jupiter
Knowledge

Ether
Mercury
Intuition

Earth
Ego
Happiness

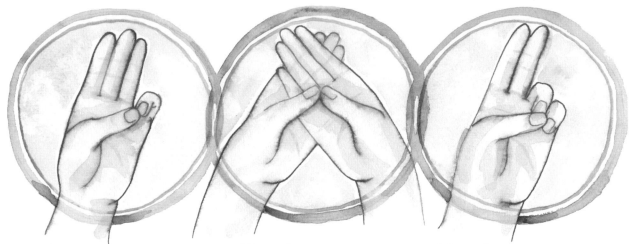

Buddhi Mudra

Join the tip of your little finger to the thumb. This links the energy of Mercury to the Earth, to foster communication and healing.

Buddha Mudra

For women, rest the left hand in the right hand. For men, the right hand rests in the left. The index fingers cross at right-angles at the upper knuckle. The thumbtips touch each other. This generates balance in the hemispheres that access the neutral mind.

Christ Mudra

Bend the little and ring fingers on to the palm and lock them there with the thumb. Extend the index and middle fingers. This balances the energy of Water and Fire.

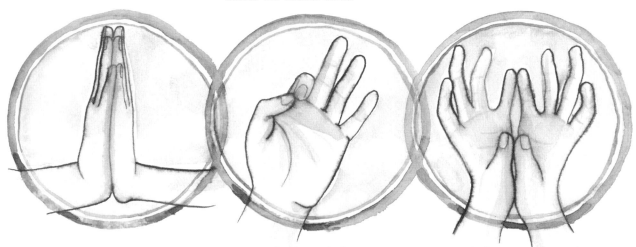

Prayer Pose Mudra

Press your palms together in the center of your chest at your heart to neutralize the positive and negative energies of the two hemispheres of the brain. Ensure that your thumbs are vertical and touch the sternum. Push the elbows forwards slightly to increase the pressure at your palms.

Gyan Mudra (receptive)

Join the tip of the index finger to the tip of the thumb, which represents the ego. This links the energy of Jupiter to the Earth to generate Divine wisdom and expansion. The active Gyan Mudra is formed by curling the nail tip of the index finger under the joint of the thumb.

Lotus Mudra

Place the heels of the hands together and join the little fingertips and the sides of the thumbs. Then spread the other fingers wide to make an inverted cone shape. This mudra is often placed at the heart, throat, or Third Eye and balances the five tattvas of the conscious and subconscious mind.

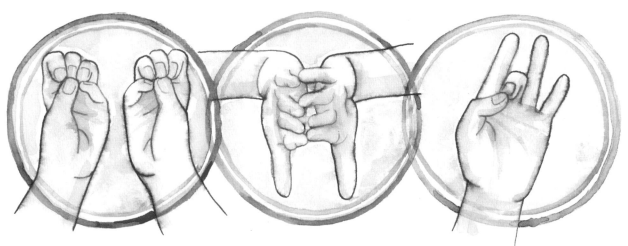

Praying Mantis Mudra
Join the tips of all fingers to the tip of the thumb to focus and blend the five elements in harmony.

Reverse Prayer Mudra (variation)
Place the hands back to back about 15 cm (6 in) just below throat level. The thumbs point down, parallel to each other. Ensure that the knuckles touch and the forearms are horizontal. This projective mudra balances the positive and negative minds.

Shuni Mudra
Join the tip of the middle finger to the thumb, representing the ego. This links the energy of Saturn to the Earth, to generate patience.

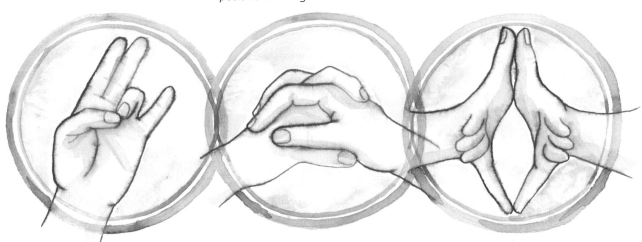

Surya Mudra
Join the tip of the ring finger to the thumb. This links the energy of the Sun to the Earth to generate powerful energy of vibrant constancy.

Venus Lock
Women interlace the fingers with the right little finger on the bottom and the left thumb on top, while men have the left little finger on the bottom and the right thumb on top. Ensure that the top thumb touches the mound of Venus on the opposite hand.

Yoni Mudra
The tips of the little fingers touch and point forwards, the sides of the thumbs touch and arch back towards the chest. The other fingers are parallel to the Earth and to each other and as far apart as possible. This tantric mudra blends the male and female polarities.

Asanas

Asanas are the body positions of yoga. There are 84 positions, or postures, which form the core practice of Hatha Yoga, the practice most commonly identified in the West as "yoga". It is said that we are all already yogis because we perform the 84 postures in the womb before birth. Holding a posture stimulates the body systems to harmonize and to heal. The postures apply subtle pressure on the glandular and nervous systems to alter the flow of energy in the nadis.

Kundalini Yoga is taught in dynamic sets, or kriyas, rather than static asanas; nevertheless we feel it is helpful to comment on some of the components of the kriyas as practicing a particular asana may help you master a kriya.

The following eighteen asanas (pp.128–33) are used in this book. Please note that different traditions name various asanas differently; for example Triangle Pose in Kundalini Yoga is called Downward-Facing Dog in Ashtanga Yoga and in Hatha Yoga Triangle Pose describes a different posture altogether.

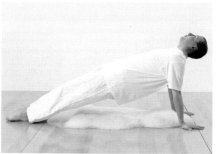

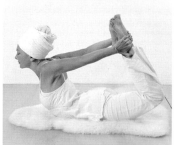

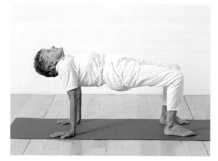

Back Platform

Sit with legs together, supporting yourself on outstretched arms behind, fingers pointing away. Inhale and raise your body until it forms a straight line (ankles, knees, hips, shoulders), from your pointed toes to your head, which is in line with your spine. Apply the Jalandhara Bandh, or Neck Lock (see p.135) and keep your shoulders relaxed.

• This strengthens your kidneys and your spine.

Bow Pose

Begin by lying on your stomach, forehead on the ground. Hold your ankles. Inhale and slowly raise your head, chest, and knees as high as you can, pointing your toes. The body will begin to rock back and forth on the Navel Point as you breathe.

• This adjusts the spine and relaxes the internal organs.

Bridge Pose

Sit on the ground and lean back on your arms, elbows locked. Bend your knees and place your feet near your buttocks. Inhale and raise your hips and torso until your body, from knee to head, is parallel with the ground. Your head is aligned with your spine and your arms and calves are vertical.

• This strengthens the back and the kidneys.

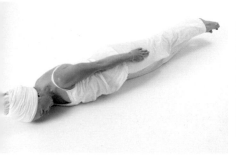

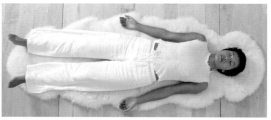

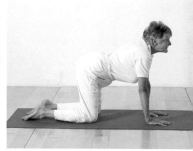

Bundle Roll

Do this dynamic asana on a soft surface. Lie on your back, heels together, arms by your sides. Tense your body as if your legs were tied together and your arms were bound to your torso. Thrust one side of the body up and begin to flip yourself over and over. Keep your arms and legs locked. The initial motion is generated from the pelvis; once created the momentum is easier to sustain. Roll in both directions.

• Balances the electromagnetic system and relaxes the nervous system, allowing it to discharge stress.

Corpse Pose

Lie flat on your back, keeping your spine warm and straight. Stretch your legs out, together or slightly apart, toes turned out and arms by your sides, palms up. Balance the left and right sides of the body and ensure that your head is not tipped to one side and that your chin does not tip upwards.

• One of the most important positions in yoga; allowing the body time to rest after the dynamic process of transformation.

Cow Pose

Come on to all fours, knees on the ground below the hips and palms on the ground beneath the shoulders. Bring the head up, turn the eyes up and look at the sky. Allow the spine to sag and the belly to drop.

• Excellent for the digestion. Builds the quality of patience.

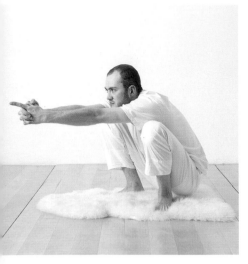

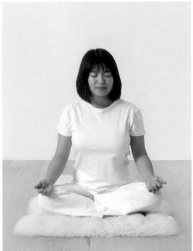

Crow Pose

*Begin standing. Gently bend the
knees and lower the hips until you
are squatting between your legs,
feet flat on the ground. Straighten
your arms and with elbows locked
interlace the fingers with the left
little finger at the bottom and the
first fingers extended. The arms
are parallel to the ground and
fully extended.*

• Balances the energy of
the First Chakra.

Easy Pose

*This basic sitting position requires
the legs to be crossed and the
spine to be straight, with
Jalandhara Bandh, or Neck Lock
(see p.135), applied. If you are
going to be sitting for any length
of time use a firm cushion to
ensure that your hips are higher
than your knees.*

Frog Pose

*Squat on the balls of the feet,
heels together and off the ground;
the hands are on the ground in
front of you. As you inhale,
straighten the legs, keeping your
heels off the ground. Exhale, bending the knees and straightening the
spine. Continue at a dynamic pace.*

• Excellent for channelling your
sexual creative energy.

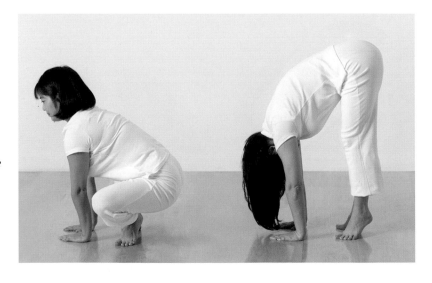

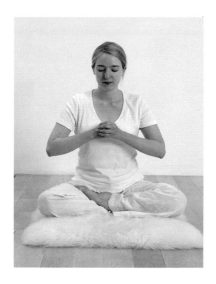

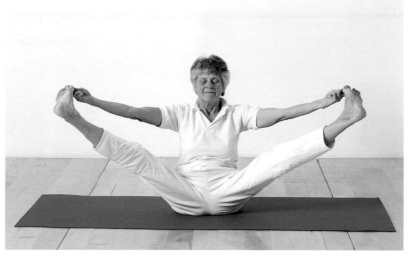

Half Lotus

This alternative sitting pose is performed by sitting cross-legged, with one foot on the opposite thigh. The other foot remains on the ground. Keep your spine straight.

Kundalini Lotus

From the sitting position, take the big toe of each foot with the thumb and first two fingers of each hand. Straighten your legs to 60 degrees to the floor and 60 degrees apart. Your spine is straight and should make a 60-degree angle with the ground.

• Excellent for balancing the Second and Sixth Chakras. Builds potency and channels the sexual energy.

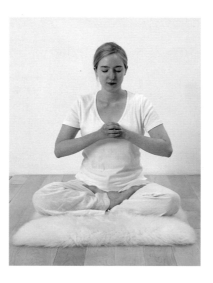

Lotus Pose

This is ideal for meditating as it offers a firm foundation and contains the energy that has been generated very effectively. Sit cross-legged, left foot on your right thigh and right foot on left thigh. Your knees should be on the ground and your spine straight. Alternate the top and bottom leg.

• Do not try to force this position. It is natural for some; others need years of practice.

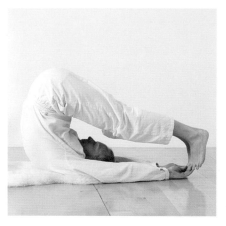

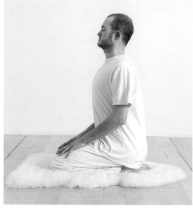

Plough Pose

Lie on your back, hands by your sides, palms down. Push down with your hands and lift your legs, bending your knees, until they are above your shoulders. Support your back with your hands so your body weight is on the shoulders, upper arms, and neck. Straighten your legs vertically by walking your hands up your spine. Now slowly lower your legs, together, over your head, until your feet touch the ground. Hold your toes and straighten your legs. A beginners' variation is to place a low chair behind to rest your legs on. Come out of the posture by supporting your back, bending your knees, and slowly unrolling into Corpse Pose (see p.129). Keep your neck straight throughout.

• Stretches the sciatic nerve, releases the spine, and flushes the head centers with blood.

Rock Pose

Sit on your heels, spine straight, with the tops of your feet on the ground. Have your palms resting comfortably on your thighs. This pose is so named because it is the best posture in which to digest anything — even rocks.

Stretch Pose

Lie on your back, arms at your sides, heels together. Lift your head, legs, arms, and heels 15 cm (6 in). Keep your toes pointed, your hands palms-down. Have your eyes open, looking at your toes. Do not arch your back. If this happens, continue, but bend the knees until your spine is straight, and then extend your legs as much as you can.

• This is a master exercise in Kundalini Yoga and essential to center the Navel Point. The Third Chakra is your physical center of gravity and focus of your personal process. This pose cleanses, detoxifies, and builds stamina.

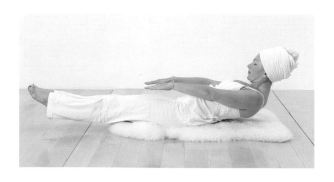

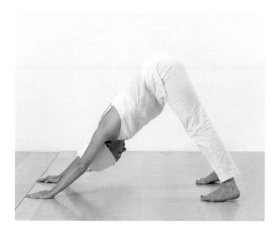

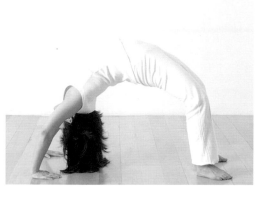

Triangle Pose

Begin on all fours and then straighten the legs until your knees are locked and your soles are on the ground. Your arms are also straight, elbows locked. The base of your spine is the apex of the triangle; one side runs from the heels to buttocks and the other along the arms and spine.

• Benefits the nervous system.

Wheel Pose

Lie on your back, bend your knees, and bring your heels to your buttocks, feet remaining flat on the ground. Bend your elbows and place your hands next to your head, on the ground, fingers pointing to your shoulders. As you inhale raise your body slowly into a wheel shape. A beginners' variation is to hold your ankles, keeping your shoulders on the ground, and push the hips as high as possible.

• Balances the flow of cerebrospinal fluid and stimulates the metabolism.

Yoga Mudra

Sit on your heels, interlacing your hands behind you in Venus Lock (see p.127) and lock your arms straight. Bring your forehead to the ground and raise your hands high.

• Stimulates and harmonizes the secretion of the thyroid, the parathyroid, the pineal, and the pituitary glands.

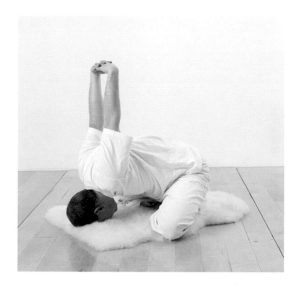

Bandhs

The science of yoga accesses the pranic Life Force and then focuses it for maximum effect before projecting or leading it to the required part of the biosystem, using "locks", or bandhs. A lock is when a defined combination of muscles is contracted, focused, and the energy appropriately projected. There are three locks that are an essential part of this process: Mul Bandh, Uddiyana Bandh, and Jalandhara Bandh. When these three are applied together they become Maha Bandh. The bandhs help to direct the flow of prana, calibrate the flow of cerebrospinal fluid, and concentrate the effects of the previous Kundalini Yoga exercise.

Mul Bandh, or Root Lock
This lock has three distinct stages. First, you contract the anal sphincter. Second, you contract the sex organs with an upwards-drawing action. Third, bring the Navel Point back towards the spine. This lock is applied as the breath is retained, either in or out. Mul Bandh concentrates the energy of the first three chakras and directs upwardly moving prana down and downwardly moving apana upwards to the Navel Point. The fusion of these two energies creates the generative force required to uncoil the Kundalini energy at the base of the spine.

• Most commonly applied with the breath held out, but may be applied either on the inhale or exhale. It is usually applied after completion of an exercise.

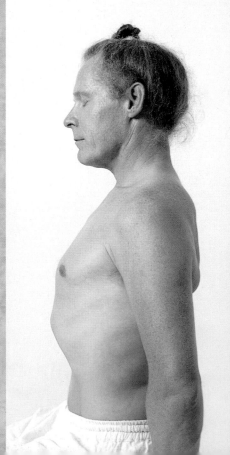

Uddiyana Bandh, or Diaphragm Lock

This lock is applied by lifting the diaphragm up and back as far into the thoracic cavity as possible and, at the same time, contracting the abdominal muscles towards the spine. This lock gently massages the intestines and heart and mediates the pranic flow through the area between the lower triangle (Mul Bandh) and the upper triangle (Jalandhara Bandh). The Diaphragm Lock is applied on the exhale. It might create pressure increases in the blood, the heart, and the eyes if applied forcefully on the inhale.

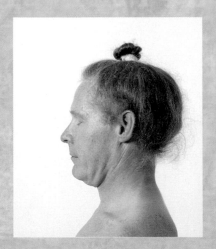

Jalandhara Bandh, or Neck Lock

The subtlest of all the locks used in Kundalini Yoga is Jalandhara Bandh, the Neck Lock. This is practiced by gently contracting on the neck and throat so that the chin settles into the notch between the two collarbones. Your head must remain level. The purpose of this lock is to align the cervical and thoracic vertebrae, allowing prana to flow into the cranial area. The psychic heat generated by Kundalini Yoga releases blocks in the nadis, which can result in dizziness. Such phenomena are minimized by an effective Jalandhara Bandh.

• An essential part of sitting with a straight spine and should be applied in all meditations and sitting asanas unless otherwise specified.

Maha Bandh

This means the Great Lock and is the name given to the application of all three locks at once. When all the locks are applied, the nervous and glandular systems are said to harmonize and the ojas (subtle fluid) is reabsorbed into the body to stimulate the higher centers as the sexual energy is channelled and absorbed.

• Effective in treating sexual dysfunctions and traditionally held to increase longevity.

Glossary

Ajna *Third Eye. Stimulated by focusing between the eyebrows at the base of the nose.*

Akashic Record *Cosmic file of all thought, deed, and intention.*

Amrit Vela *Ambrosial hours before dawn, when the devout celebrate the Divine within and without.*

Apana *The "downward breath" is the eliminative aspect of prana.*

Aquarian Age *We are currently in the cusp between the ages of Pisces and Aquarius, which begins on December 21st, 2012.*

Asana *The body positions of yoga.*

Ashtanga *Eight beats, referring to mantras with eight syllables.*

Bhakti *One filled with devotion for his God or Guru. Bhakti Yoga is recognized as an exemplary path of yoga in itself.*

Bandh *Lock. Four principal locks of Kundalini Yoga are Mul Bandh, Uddiyana Bandh, Jalandhara Bandh, and Maha Bandh.*

Bij *Seed, referring to one- or two-syllable mantras that grow in the psyche to "seed" trees of consciousness when watered by consistent spiritual practice.*

Bodhisattva *"Buddha to be", or Buddhist saint.*

Chakra *"Lotus", or "wheel"; the seven energetic vortices created where the Ida and Pingala intersect across the Sushumna.*

Dharana *Steady concentration.*

Dhyana *Contemplation.*

Golden Chain *Divine energetic link of spiritual masters connected with when chanting the Adi Mantra.*

Golden Cord *Energetic connection of Seventh to Sixth Chakra threaded through the pineal, pituitary, and hypothalamus glands.*

Gunas *Three inherent states of matter and nature: tamas, rajas, and sattva.*

Guru *Often "teacher", meaning "dark" to "light" (gu-ru); a process rather than a person embodying such a process.*

Guru Ram Das *Patron saint of Kundalini Yoga.*

Hatha Yoga *"Ha" = Sun and "tha" = Moon; hence "the union experienced when Sun and Moon channels (Ida and Pingala) harmonize".*

Heart Center *Point of focus at the center of the chest, corresponding to the Heart Chakra.*

Higher Self *Soul-consciousness relating to the upper chakras.*

Ida *A major nadi. Coils around Sushumna and carries the female lunar current through left nostril.*

Jnana *Self-knowledge*

Kabbalah *Ancient spiritual system, taught by Moses to the Jews, and by the Gnostic Christians.*

Karma *Law of cause and effect.*

Kirtan *Sacred music and chanting; central to Sikh Dharma and Sufism, where chanting stimulates the correct sequence of pressure points on the upper palate, generating heightened awareness.*

Kriya *Completed action: the combined effect of the mudra, mantra, asana, breath, and bandh contained in the sequence of exercises. Hence, "Kriya for Elevation" or "Kriya to open the Heart Chakra". But a kriya may comprise one single practice, e.g. "Sat Kriya".*

Kundalini *Literally, the Curl of the Hair of the Beloved. Kundalini is the latent creative potential of the human being, which when dormant, lies coiled at the base of the spine.*

Laya Yoga *Applied science of sound, rhythm, and locks. An integral part of Kundalini Yoga.*

Logos *Divine Word as perceived by the ancient adepts.*

Mahan Tantric *Mantle of the Master of White Tantric Yoga.*

Mantra *Word or sound that sets subtle energies in vibration. Used in meditations.*

MEDITATION *Establishment of an internal dialogue with the Divine.*

MERIDIANS *Channels of subtle energy, common to Eastern practices such as acupuncture and shiatsu.*

MUDRA *Hand position. Many Kundalini kriyas specify a mudra.*

NADI *Channels of subtle energy within the body.*

NAM *Name of God or the resonance of totality. By repeating the Nam, the aspirant merges with, and finally embodies, the One.*

NAVEL POINT *50 mm (2 in) below the umbilicum, a major intersection of energetic channels in the body, starting point of the 72,000 nadis corresponding to the Third Chakra.*

NIYAMAS *"Five yogic observances" to which the yogic aspirant should adhere: purity, contentment, austerity, study, and recognition of the One.*

OJAS *Subtlest refined essence of the cerebrospinal fluid.*

PARVATI *The first yoga student; consort of, and complement to, Shiva. Represents Shakti power.*

PINGALA *Major nadi coiled around the Sushumna carrying the male solar current through the right nostril.*

PISCEAN AGE *Period ending on December 21st, 2012.*

PRANA *The Life Force. Named qi, chi, or ki in other traditions.*

PRANAYAMA *Literally to "lead the Life Force". Refers to the science of yogic breath control.*

PRATYAHARA *"Withdrawal of the senses".*

QAWWALI *Literally "the mouthpiece of Divine power"; the sacred hymns of the Sufis.*

RAJ YOGA *The Royal Path or the yoga of mastery of the mind.*

RAJAS *Activity, creativity, and the kinetic principle.*

SADHANA *Spiritual practice especially during the amrit vela.*

SADHU *Yogi or yogini who has established a powerful spiritual practice, or "Sadhana".*

SAMADHI *State of self-realization; complete absorption within the Infinite.*

SANSKRIT *Earliest-known Indo-European language.*

SAT YUG *Golden Age of Truth, in which peace, harmony, and elevated spiritual consciousness prevailed.*

SATTVA *One of the three conditions of matter, denoting purity and illumination.*

SHAKTI *Creative power of Shiva, the feminine creative principle.*

SHIVA *Lord of Yoga, destroyer and creator, embodies the eternal paradox; represents the male principle.*

SILVER CORD *Energetic pathway from the base of the spine to the pituitary gland, or Sixth Chakra.*

SUFISM *Energetic inner heart of Islamic practice.*

SUSHUMNA *Central spine of chakra system: vertical nadi by which Kundalini ascends.*

TAMAS *One of the three conditions of matter, characterized by decay and inertia.*

TANTRA *"Length and breadth", the yogic science of expanding the parameters of the subtle energetic body and the psyche.*

TATTVAS *All phenomena in the Universe are comprised of the five elements: Ether, Air, Fire, Water, and Earth.*

THIRD EYE POINT *A point of focus at the center of the brow, corresponding to the Sixth Chakra.*

VEDAS *Sacred texts compiled in India during the Vedic Period 3000 years ago.*

YAMAS *Five yogic abstinences: non-violence, truthfulness, not stealing, continence, and not being greedy.*

Bibliography and resources

Please note that only Kundalini Yoga manuals with the Kundalini Research Institute (KRI) Seal of Approval contain authenticated kriyas and meditations as taught by Yogi Bhajan.

Some of the following books and products may be temporarily unavailable or out of print. You may be able to find these at www.kundaliniyoga.org or obtain one from one of the resources listed on p.139. You can also try your library or secondhand bookstore.

KUNDALINI YOGA:
SADHANA GUIDELINES, Arcline/KRI, 1988
The original beginners' guide to Kundalini Yoga — the teachings of Yogi Bhajan, compiled by Gurucharan Singh Khalsa

MEDITATION MANUAL FOR INTERMEDIATE STUDENTS, KRI, 1976
A rich compendium of Kundalini Yoga kriyas and meditations, compiled by Gurucharan Singh Khalsa

THE TEACHINGS OF YOGI BHAJAN, Hawthorn, 1977
A unique, essential transmission

THE MASTER'S TOUCH, KRI, 1997
An illuminating transcription of two courses taught by Yogi Bhajan in 1996. The next best thing to being there and including all the meditations given

Kaur Khalsa, Shakta, KUNDALINI YOGA, Dorling Kindersley, 2000

CHAKRAS
Hetzel, Rattana Ph.D (aka Guru Rattan Kaur Khalsa), YOUR LIFE IS IN YOUR CHAKRAS, Yoga Technology Press, 1994

Judith, Anodea, WHEELS OF LIFE, Llewellyn, 1988

Leadbeater, CW, THE CHAKRAS, Theosophical, 1972 (Quest, 1974)

Wilson, A & Beck, L, WHAT COLOUR ARE YOU?, Aquarian Press, 1981

YOGIC NUMEROLOGY
Khalsa, Guruchander S, TANTRIC NUMEROLOGY, Radiant Light, 1992

Khalsa, Guruchander S, NUMEROLOGY, Radiant Light, 1992

Singh, Ravi, COUNT YOUR BLESSINGS, White Lion, 1994

YOGIC DIET
THE GOLDEN TEMPLE VEGETARIAN COOKBOOK, Arcline, 1978

Sivananda Center, THE YOGA COOKBOOK, Fireside, 1999

Siri Amir Singh Khalsa, FOODS FOR HEALTH AND HEALING, available from (800) 359-2940 or www.a-healing.com

GENERAL
Avalon, Arthur, THE SERPENT POWER, Dover, 1974

Bahm, Archie J, THE YOGA SUTRAS OF PATANJALI, Jain, 1993

Burger, Bruce, ESOTERIC ANATOMY, North Atlantic, 1998

Fraser, JG, THE GOLDEN BOUGH, Simon and Schuster, 1996

Gerber, R, A PRACTICAL GUIDE TO VIBRATIONAL MEDICINE, Quill, 2001

Johari, Harish, LEELA, Destiny, 1980

Mookerjee, Ajit, KUNDALINI THE AROUSAL OF INNER ENERGY, Inner Traditions, 1982

Waterstone, Richard, INDIA, Thorsons, 1995

Yatri, UNKNOWN MAN, Sidgwick & Jackson, 1988

MUSIC AND MANTRA FOR YOGA AND MEDITATION
COMPANION CD TO THE KUNDALINI YOGA EXPERIENCE, by various artists, www.mayarecords.co.uk

These are some of the authors' other favorites for yogic practice and deep relaxation:

THE GONG NAMO
by Guru Dharam
www.72bpm.org

RA MA DA SA SA SAY SO HUNG
by Gurnaam Rootlight Inc.
CD 9901TM

TRIPLE MANTRA
by Gurnaam Rootlight Inc.
Performed by Gurunam, orchestra by Torkel Berg, CD 9902RA

THE CRIMSON SERIES
by Singh Kaur
Invincible Productions
INV 308, 309, 310

JAP MAN SAT NAM
by Guru Raj Kaur Khalsa
GRD Recordings

NARAYAN
by Guru Raj Kaur Khalsa
GRD Recordings

WHA HE GURU JIO
by Giani Ji
Invincible Productions

TANTRIC HAR and TANTRIC MOOL MANTRA
by Simran Kaur
Cherdi Kala Music

Certified Training in Kundalini Yoga
SKY The School of Kundalini Yoga
34 Culver Road
Newbury
Berkshire
RG14 7AR
United Kingdom
TEL: 00 44 (0) 1635 523900
FAX: (760) 923-9514
EMAIL: sky@i-sky.net
WEB: www.i-sky.net

Courses, Classes, Consultations
Darryl O'Keeffe
Contact via SKY, details as above

Guru Dharam Singh Khalsa
Studio 163
3 Edgar Buildings
George Street
Bath
BA1 2FJ
United Kingdom
TEL: 00 44 (0) 7958 928252
EMAIL: gdskyoga@btinternet.com
WEB: www.72bpm.org

Kundalini Yoga Teachers Associations
To find a Kundalini Yoga center or
teacher in your area contact:
IKYTA the International Kundalini
Yoga Teachers Association
TEL: (505) 367-1313
FAX: (505) 753-1999
EMAIL: ikyta@3ho.org
WEB: www.kundaliniyoga.com

Yogi Bhajan and 3HO, the Healthy Happy Holy Organisation
3Ho
6 Narayan Court
Espanola
NM 87532, USA
TEL: (888) 346-2420, (505) 367-1326
FAX: (505) 753-1999
EMAIL: yogainfo@3ho.org
WEB: www.3ho.org

Other Resources
Ancient Healing Ways
PO Box 130
Espanola
NM 87532, USA
TEL: (505) 747-2860
FAX: (505) 747-2868
*For a catalog call (800) 359-2940,
or visit www.a-healing.com.*

Cherdi Kala Catalog
436 N. Bedford Drive
Suite 308
Beverly Hills, CA 90210
Tel/Fax: (310) 838-9989
WEB: www.cherdikala.com
Books, videos, audiotapes and CDs

Golden Temple Enterprises
Box 13
Shady Lane
Espanola
NM 87532, USA
TEL: (505) 753-0563
Fax: (505) 753-5603
WEB: www.goldentempleusa.com
(800) 829-3970
*Video & audiotapes of Yogi
Bhajan's classes*

Invincible Recordings
PO. Box 13054
Phoenix
AZ 85002, USA
TEL: (800) 829-3970
WEB: www.invinciblemusic.com
Audio tapes and CDs

Rootlight, Inc
PO Box 7945
New York
NY 10116-7945, USA
TEL/FAX: (212) 769-8115
WEB: www.rootlight.com
Audio tapes and CDs

Instruction tape for energy healing
MIND THE GAP BY Darryl O'Keeffe &
Shirley Brooker
Available from NFSH the National
Federation of Spiritual Healers
Old Manor Farm Studio
Church Street
Sunbury on Thames
Middlesex TW16 6RG, UK
TEL: 01932 783164
FAX: 01932 779648
EMAIL: office@nfsh.org.uk
WEB: www.nfsh.org.uk

About the authors

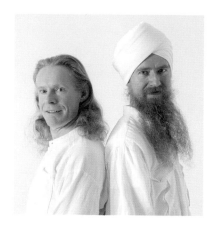

Darryl O'Keeffe *qualified as a teacher while attending the Central School of Speech and Drama in London and he has practiced as a part-time teacher since 1978. Initially his employment took him from fringe theater, through community theater, to director of a youth and community center.*
In the early 1980s he began to "catch" other people's headaches and discovered that he could physically remove pain from other people. His spiritual reawakening began consciously when he took a migraine away from a girlfriend in the street. The energetic discharge knocked him over and rendered him unconscious for a moment and as he lay there contemplating the stars, he mused that what had just happened was impossible by any science that he had ever been taught. At that moment he resolved to find out what was really going on in the world. His enquiries led him to the National Federation of Spiritual Healers and by the late 1980s he had become a practicing spiritual healer and was teaching others. After attending a Kundalini healing course with Lilla Bek he started adopting yoga postures during his meditation practice. He began to practice yoga, joining three classes: Hatha, Iyengar, and Kundalini. Although he maintained his Hatha yoga practice for several years it was the spiritual dimension of the Kundalini Yoga classes taught by Guru Dharam Singh Khalsa that really resonated with him. Darryl is a much-traveled and practically minded spiritual teacher and healer, registered as a Teacher

Trainer with the International Kundalini Yoga Teachers Association and teaches holistic healing for a variety of organizations including the National Federation of Spiritual Healers, the School of Insight and Intuition, and several, more conventional, educational establishments. He has taught all over the world and conducts SAcred Tours to a number of countries with his friend and mentor Judy Fraser of www.Second Aid.net. He has recorded several audiotapes of an instructional and meditative nature and has made a variety of television, radio, and press contributions. Darryl teaches regularly and maintains a consultative yoga and healing practice.

Guru Dharam Singh Khalsa *was born in London of Yorkshire and Russian parentage. He encountered Kundalini Yoga one day in 1981 and began a daily practice the next. He met the Siri Singh Sahib Yogi Bhajan in 1982 and started teaching Kundalini Yoga. Over the years he developed a practice in Kundalini therapeutics and was inspired to learn Oriental energetic medicine. Formal study resulted in qualifications as an acupuncturist*

in 1989 and as a herbalist in 1991, completing his post-graduate clinical study in Ho Chi Min City. He founded the Lotus Healing Centre in 1989 and served as the Vice Principal of the London Academy of Oriental Medicine until 1996. A fascination with the phenomenon and presence of the gong, mantra, and healing circles of his Kundalini practice led to his pioneering work in the development of Sahaj Sound, a sonic therapeutic healing modality for the 21st century. He is currently developing the clinical usage of Electronic Gem Lamp Therapy, a modern application of the ancient science of healing with gemstones. Study of the Kabbalah and the meso-American indigenous practice of Awakened Dreaming provide continued energetic and professional development alongside his first love, Kundalini Yoga. Guru Dharam was the first chairperson of the Kundalini Yoga Teachers Association in the UK and is registered as a Teacher Trainer with the International Kundalini Yoga Teachers Association. He facilitates contemporary applications of ancient healing techniques and teaches Kundalini Yoga around the world. Guru Dharam lives in London, where he has an established medical practice.

Guru Dharam and Darryl established SKY, the School of Kundalini Yoga, in 1996; like their teacher Yogi Bhajan before them, they are teaching for the Aquarian Age, teaching others how to practice and instruct the sacred art and science that is Kundalini Yoga.

Index

Main entries are in **bold**. See also Glossary.

1st Chakra–7th Chakra *see individual entries* First Chakra–Seventh Chakra

Adi Mantra 52, **53**, **122**
Ajna *see* Sixth Chakra
all is one 17
Anahata *see* Fourth Chakra
Arc Line (yogic body 6) 17, 18, **26**
    meditation (6a, 6b) 111
as above so below 125
asanas **128–35**
Aura (yogic body 7) 17, 18, **27**
    meditation (7a, 7b) 112

Back Platform 128
balance 24, 25, 73
Base Chakra *see* First Chakra
bandhs 14, **134–5**
bij (seed) mantras 121
birth dates 17
bodies *see* yogic bodies
body locks *see* bandhs
Bow Pose 128
brain 95, 109
breath/breathing **28**, 52, 56, **119–20**
    alternate nostril breathing **120**
    and brainwave patterns 119
    deep 84
    long, deep breathing **119**
    paradoxically 120
Breath of Fire **120**
Bridge Pose 128
Buddha Mudra 126
Buddhi Mudra 126
Bundle Roll 129
Butterfly 55

Cat Stretch 57
cautions 8, 9
cerebrospinal fluid 134
chakras 11, 14, **32–4**, **35–41**

and physical body **34**
    balance **42**
    blocked/unblocked 42
    correspondences 33, **35–41**
    open/closed 42
    questionnaire 42, **43–9**
    using 34
    see also individual chakras (First–Seventh)
Christ Mudra 126
clothing 9, 52
colours 33
Completion 58–9
consciousness 14, 31, 32
Corpse Pose 129
cosy and contented 115
Cow Pose 129
creative impulses 90
Crow Pose 130
Crown Chakra *see* Seventh Chakra

Deep Relaxation 57
depression 83, 107, 108
Destiny Number 17, **20**
Diaphragm Lock *see* Uddiyana Bandh
digestion 66, 83, 102
Divine 12, 21, 111
do your best 9
duality 22

Easy Pose 130
ecstasy 117
ego 108, 109, 125
Ego Eradicator 56
electromagnetic energy/field 17, 27, 52
elements 95, 125
elimination 66
Embodiment (yogic body 11) 18, **31**
    meditation (11a, 11b) 116–17
endocrine glands 32, **34**, 93, 102
energy healing 32
enthusiasm 23
equilibrium 31

evolution, process of 32
fear 112, 113
feel good 84
Fifth Chakra (5th; Throat Chakra) 32, 34, **39**
    kriya (5a) 88–90, 5b (91–3)
    questionnaire 47
First Chakra (1st; Root or Base Chakra) 14, 32, 34, **35**
    kriya (1a) 64–6, (1b) 67–9
    questionnaire 43
Fourth Chakra (4th; Heart Center) 32, 34, **38**
    kriya (4a) 84, (4b) 85–7
    questionnaire 46
foundation on Earth 105
Frog Pose 130
future, insight of the 111

Gift Number 17, **20**
God **8**, 11, 31
Gyan Mudra 126

Half Lotus 131
Hatha Yoga 12, 128
Heart Center *see* Fourth Chakra

I am, I am 110, 124
Infinity 28, 31
intuition 102

Jalandhara Bandh, or Neck Lock 52, **135**

Karma Number 17, **19**
Kirtan Kriya Meditation 58, **62**, 63
kriyas 42, 56, 65, **64–105**
    every day (Sat Kriya) **61**
    length of time to practice 51
Kundalini 11, **12**, 14
Kundalini Lotus 131
Kundalini Yoga 8, 11, 32, **51**
    environment 52
    established, safe practice 51, **52**
    Kriya 56, **61**

length of practice 51
Meditation 58, **62**
personal preparation 52
time of day to practice **52**

Laya Yoga 11–12
Leg and Torso Stretch 55
Leg Stretch 55
life path 18
Light 30, 33
locks *see* bandhs
Lotus Mudra 126
Lotus Pose 131
lower chakras 32, 33, 42

Maha Bandh 135
Manipura *see* Third Chakra
mantras 13, 110, **121–4**
    and Tuning Out 59
    and Warm-Up Exercises 54
    English-language 124
    pronunciation guide 121
meditations 58, **106–17**
    every day (Kirtan Kriya) **62**
meditative mind 109
memories 27
menstruation 9
mind 17, 90
mudras **125–7**
Mul Bandh, or Root Lock 14, 52,
    134
Muladhara *see* First Chakra

Navel Chakra *see* Third Chakra
Navel Point 14
Neck Lock *see* Jalandhara Bandh
negative 108
Negative Mind (yogic body 2) 17,
    18, **22**
    meditation (2a, 2b) 107
nervous plexus 32, 34
Neutral Mind (yogic body 4) 17, 18,
    24
    meditation (4a, 4b) 109
numerology, numbers, yogic *see*

yogic numerology

One 31

Path Number 17, **20**
Physical Body (yogic body 5) 17, 18,
    25
    meditation (5a, 5b) 110
Plough Pose 132
positive 108
Positive Mind (yogic body 3) 17, 18,
    23
    meditation (3a, 3b) 108
prana 17, 27, 28, **119**
    and bandhs (locks) 134
pranayama 84, **119**
Pranic Body (yogic body 8) 17, 18,
    28
    meditation (8a, 8b) 113
Prayer Pose 126
Praying Mantis Mudra 127
pregnancy 9
project, projections 26
psyche 17, 125

radiance 18, 30, 115
Radiant Body (yogic body 10) 18,
    30
    meditation (10a, 10b) 115
relaxation 112
Reverse Prayer Mudra 127
Rock Pose 132
Root Chakra *see* First Chakra
Root Lock *see* Mul Bandh

Sa Ta Na Ma **62**, 63, 123
Sacral Chakra *see* Second Chakra
safe practice 51, 52
Sahasrara *see* Seventh Chakra
Samadhi **13**
Sanskrit 121
Sat Kriya 56, **61**
Sat Nam 54, **59**, 99, 107, 123
Second Chakra (2nd; Sacral Chakra)
    32, 34, **36**

kriya (2a) 70–3, (2b) 74–7
questionnaire 44
serpent 12
Seventh Chakra (7th; Crown Chakra)
    14, 32, 34, **41**
    kriya (7a) 100–2, (7b) 103–5
    questionnaire 49
sexual system/energy 61, 102
Shiva 11, 14
Shuni Mudra 127
Siri Gaitri Mantra 123
Sixth Chakra (6th; Third Eye) 32,
    34, **40**
    kriya (6a) 94–5, (6b) 96–9
    questionnaire 48
soul 17, 18, 19, 21
Soul Body (yogic body 1) 17, 18, **21**
    meditation (1a, 1b) 106
Soul Number 17, **19**
Spinal Flex (1, 2, 3) 53–4
Spinal Twist 54
spine, flexibility of 66
spiritual technology 11, 17
Stretch Pose 132
subconscious 29, 117
subtle bodies 18
Subtle Body (yogic body 9) 17, 18,
    29
    meditation (9a, 9b) 114
Surya Mudra 127
Svadhisthana *see* Second Chakra

Tantra Yoga 11, 12
Third Chakra (3rd; Navel Chakra)
    32, 34, **37**
    kriya (3a) 78–80, (3b) 81–3
    questionnaire 45
Third Eye *see* Sixth Chakra
Throat Chakra *see* Fifth Chakra
tongue, position of 121
Triangle Pose 133
truth 19, 110
Tune In 53

Uddiyana Bandh, or Diaphragm

Lock 14, **135**
unfold 112
upper chakras 32, 42
Venus Lock 127
vibrations 17, 33, 42
Virasan 94
Vishuddha *see* Fifth Chakra
Wake-Up Sequence 57
Warm Up 52, **53–6**
well-being 110
Wheel Pose 133
women, special note 9, 105
yoga 11
   body positions *see* asanas
   eight limbs 11
   hand gestures *see* mudras
   nine modern paths 12
   three original forms 11, 12
Yoga Mudra 133
Yogi Bhajan 15
yogic bodies **17–18**
yogic numerology **17–20**
yoni 114
Yoni Mudra 127

ACKNOWLEDGEMENTS

Gaia Books would like to thank the following for their help in the creation of this book: Jenny and Owen Dixon and Mark Preston for design assistance; Lynn Bresler for proofreading and indexing; Bridget Lytton Minor, Elena O'Keeffe, Emna Diamant, Garz Chan, Jae Charles, Joy Tadaki, Julie Cuddihy, Matt Jones, Nidhan Kaur, Owain James, Pat Postle, Pavllou Landraagon, Rafael Ramos and Rob Alcock for modelling; Satya Kaur Khalsa and her colleagues at the Kundalini Research Institute (KRI), and Pip Morgan for editorial development.

The authors would like to humbly thank: Yogi Bhajan and the Golden Chain which passes now from the Infinite One through yourself and which links us all as students to our teachers and as teachers to our students.

At the time of publication KRI have been unable confirm the accuracy of three meditations (see pp 74, 113 and 114) sourced from original student transcriptions of Yogi Bhajan's classes. The authors believe the instructions to be accurate but for details of any corrections subsequently requested by KRI please go to
http://www.i-sky.net